Pragmatic Children's Nursing

Pragmatic Children's Nursing is the first attempt to create a paedi-atric nursing theory which argues for the importance of giving children living with illness access to a childhood which is, as far as possible, equal to that of their peers. Set in the historical context of the development of children's nursing, this theory is presented in detail as an educational process, complete with eight outcome measures which allow the practitioner to evaluate its effectiveness.

In this book Randall explores the triad relationship between children, carers and nurses within the context of healthcare delivery. He analyses the moral and ethical implications of pragmatic children's nursing, which challenges the established ideas of family-centred care. In addition to offering theoretical grounding and debate, Randall presents four practical case studies which model how this theory may work within various hospital and community settings.

Establishing a link between the concepts inherent in pragmatism and our understanding of childhood within society, this acces-sible book will appeal to a global audience of undergraduate and postgraduate nursing students, researchers and policy makers.

Duncan C. Randall is a Principal Teaching Fellow in Health Sciences at the University of Southampton.

Routledge Research in Nursing

1 Pragmatic Children's Nursing
A theory for children and their childhoods
Duncan C. Randall

Pragmatic Children's Nursing

A theory for children and their childhoods

Duncan C. Randall

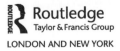

Routledge
Taylor & Francis Group

LONDON AND NEW YORK

First published 2016
by Routledge
2 Park Square, Milton Park, Abingdon, Oxon OX14 4RN

and by Routledge
711 Third Avenue, New York, NY 10017

First issued in paperback 2017

Routledge is an imprint of the Taylor & Francis Group, an informa business

British Library Cataloguing in Publication Data
A catalogue record for this book is available from the British Library

Library of Congress Cataloging in Publication Data
Randall, Duncan C., author.
Pragmatic children's nursing : a theory for children and their childhoods / Duncan C. Randall.
p. ; cm. -- (Routledge research in nursing)
Includes bibliographical references and index.
I. Title. II. Series: Routledge research in nursing.
[DNLM: 1. Pediatric Nursing--methods. 2. Nurse-Patient Relations. 3. Nursing Theory. 4. Parent-Child Relations. 5. Professional-Family Relations. WY 159]
RJ245
618.92'00231--dc23
2015012126

ISBN: 978-1-138-55293-7 (pbk)
ISBN: 978-1-138-89806-6 (hbk)

Typeset in Sabon
by Fakenham Prepress Solutions, Fakenham, Norfolk NR21 8NN

Contents

Preface

My purpose here is to set out my understanding of the theories which inform, shape and limit the practice of children's nursing. I will try to avoid the overblown language which is often employed in the discussion of ethics, philosophy and theoretical nursing. For no other reason other than my belief that understanding the theories which nurses employ will help them deliver care to children. My intention is not to dress these theoretical understandings in language and constructions which require years of study, by elite scholars, to be understood, but to speak as plainly as I can to nurses who work with children and their carers. Because it is the right of every child to receive healthcare and the duty of all nurses to share their understanding and skills to enable children to receive such care.

The impetus to write this text came from working with students over a number of years exploring the theoretical basis of children's nursing. I have to thank the many students who helped to inform and shape my thinking by challenging my assumptions. The problem, which occurred each year, when we did the session on children's nursing theory, was that the textbook nursing theories assumed the client/patient is a cognisant adult. None of them incorporated our concerns as children's nurses for the child, for childhoods to be lived, or for parents trying to parent children living with illness. Thus this attempt to construct a theoretical approach to children's nursing which would account for childhood as a part of the structure of societies.

I begin then by exploring the difficulty that adult-focused nursing theory gives to nurses working with children. I discuss the lack of models and theories which are specifically designed to account for children and their childhood. I then consider the assumptions about understanding and the moral purpose of children's nursing which underpins the theoretical approach taken. Having set out the foundations, I go on to explore the relationships between the nurse, organisations, children, parents and communities. What I propose is that nursing children in health and illness is a negotiated practice which exists within a cultural and social time and space. The moral 'good' which nursing aims to deliver can only be understood as a part of cultural, social and political practices within communities. In particular the objectives of children's nursing are a part of a community's project to nurture the next generation. As such I propose that one of the central purposes of children's nursing is to facilitate children who experience illness, live with illness or disability, or live with a life-threatening/limiting condition to have a childhood which, as far as possible, is similar to that of their peers within their communities.

This facilitation by nurses of a lived childhood for some children is directly related to two other aspects of children's nursing: one, the support of the practice of medicine; and two, the support of the practices of parenting. Children's nursing can be seen then as linking children living a childhood, being parented by their parents within their community, and medical practices which promote health, prevent or treat illness and or manage symptoms and the process of dying.

The cultural and social stance put forward here raises some challenges for children's nurses in pursuing a negotiated moral objective of delivering 'good' children's nursing. In that locating children's nursing in a cultural and social space and time may help to expose ethically questionable practice but also raises spectres of relativism and ideology.

At the end of the book I have attempted to pull all the threads together and give practical examples of how I conceive the theory, discussed here, could be put into practice.

Whether the ideas I have put forward here are useful or need revising over time is perhaps not the point. Just as in any human relationship, the point is that we have started to talk about what children's nursing is, what it aims to do and what it can give to children, their parents, families, friends and communities.

Duncan Randall
RCN library, London

A note on terms used

Children living with illness

This term is intended to include children living with disability and/or those living with a life-threatening or limiting condition, on occasion all three terms are stated but to save repetition sometimes just the term 'children living with illness' is used. Within the term, illness is used on purpose as the experience of disease. Health promotion and public health aspects of children's nursing are discussed in more detail in Chapter 2.

Children's carers

It is recognised that in the main it is mothers who are children's main carers when they live with illness, however, this term is used to include fathers, siblings, grandparents and any other family member who acts as a child's carer. Sometimes the term is followed by (parents) to emphasise that in the main parents of both genders deliver care, but it is not intended that this limit the term to just mothers and fathers.

Children's nurse

People who deliver nursing care to children as a part of their occupation. This term is not intended to be limited to nurses holding a specialist children's nursing educational qualification or category of registration.

Figures

Boxes

1 If it quacks like a pigeon, it's a duck! The context of children's nursing

Introduction

The statement in the title of this chapter – if it quacks like a pigeon, it's a duck! – is of course nonsensical. It is, however, the approach which seems to have been taken to children's nursing and healthcare. Rather than deriving theory, policy or practices on understanding what childhood is, what it feels like to be a child, traditionally healthcare for children has been based on adult healthcare. The models of nursing critiqued in this chapter have been applied to children, but none of them was derived from empirical studies with children, or from literature written about children, not even from the understanding about children of nurses or carers (parents etc.) who have worked with children. I want to argue that trying to adapt adult conceptual frameworks and nursing theories to children is not only problematic and nonsensical, but also damaging to children. In that these adult-adapted approaches do not facilitate children's access to a childhood, in effect the omission of any aspect of childhood is to suggest that children do not need to experience a childhood, to deny them access to their childhood. This denial of children's access to a childhood is a denial of their basic human right to grow and develop within a community. As Kelly et al. (2012) have pointed out, children's rights have not been well represented, or honoured in healthcare. The use of adult-adapted models would seem not to have encouraged health workers to meet the needs of children.

The review of literature undertaken by Kelly et al. (2012) uses the concept of family-centred care. Here surely is the answer, a concept outlined by Ann Cassey (1988), a children's nurse, with lots of experience of nursing children. As we shall see, even if 'family-centred care' existed beyond being a professional concept (Shields et al. 2012), or perhaps more properly a professional foundation myth (Arbuckle 2013), then conceptually it still does not account for children living a childhood.

To understand, however, why children's nursing did not develop its own theories, we need to understand first the historical background to how children's nursing developed as a separate aspect of nursing, particularly in the UK.

A critical history of children's nursing: the isolation of children in healthcare

It is not surprising that the more recent focus on children's transitions from children services to adult services has been challenging and problematic (Royal College of Nursing Adolescent Health Forum 2008; Royal College of Nursing Children and Young People's Mental Health Forum 2008), as for over 200 years children's services have been separated from those offered to adults.

Arguably the schism in children's healthcare came in the 1740s. Until this time children were cared for with their mothers, most often in the family home, occasionally with adults in monasteries or other faith-inspired institutions (Lomax 1996). Despite little attention being paid to children and their healthcare, the treatment of children prior to the establishment of paediatrics as a subspecialty in medicine was perhaps not so unfamiliar. Williams (2007) has described four cases of children treated both as inpatients and as outpatients at Northampton county voluntary hospital in 1744–45. She discusses the many similarities between the health needs of these children over two centuries ago and present health challenges, albeit that the historical record for children's healthcare is scant and that often the treatment of children has to be pieced together from details contained in more general adult-focused documents, as Williams (2007) has done from the general hospital regulations. As Williams (2007) also notes, the official documents of healthcare organisations may not give a true picture of actual practices. Elizabeth Agar, aged 8, seems to have been admitted in 1745 despite a one-month history of fever in contravention of the hospital regulation on admitting patients with infectious diseases.

Lindsay (2001) also points to the lack of research on more typical provincial hospitals and how nurses in particular may not have enacted the regulations of the institutions, often appearing to allow 'unofficial' visiting of children by their parents. Thus the historical record of children's nursing may need to be approached with some scepticism since children and women are often omitted from the records of institutions and the state, the very records which are archived and preserved. These records are easier to obtain and research, which leads to a bias in the historical analysis towards larger institutions and state records over informal sources (Lindsay 2001). In addition we cannot assume that people and nurses always respected the regulations and diktats of hospital elites.

Armed with suitable scepticism of the historical evidence, we can say that with the Enlightenment and the revolutions in France and America came ideas that childhood is a separate and important time (for details on Rousseau and Locke, see James et al. 1998) and a sufficient conception of fraternity to inspire people such as sea captain William Coram to establish orphanages. Coram was appalled on his return to London to see orphans dying on the street. This cannot have been a new phenomenon, although it may have worsened with urbanisation. To be inspired to act as Coram did, to change what he saw, required that the views of the poor and their offspring had to change, from one of the poor as deserving of their fate, due to inadequacy or sin, to one in which those living in poverty were seen as fellow humans in need of care and help. We can see this shift from the religious ideas about access to healthcare to an egalitarian ideal of equality of access by looking back to the admission process described by Williams (2007). Prior to the spread of Enlightenment ideas, children were only admitted to voluntary hospitals by recommendation of a subscriber. Those who were wealthy enough to afford the £2 per month subscription for Northampton county hospital (Williams 2007) would recommend those they felt worthy, with strong religious injunctions. Patients (or presumably the child's parents, see Lindsay 2001) were expected to be from a parish and to give thanks for their care to the parish church as well as observing religious practices and general behaviour during their treatment (Williams 2007). Contrast this with the requirement placed on Coram's foundling hospital that all children be admitted (Whitting

2005) albeit that the so-called General Reception (1756–60) was a disaster for the 10,389 children who died in those years and was replaced with an interview process when the foundling hospital reopened in 1763, and which by 1795 included an assessment of the mothers' 'moral' character and behaviour (Howell 2014). The Enlightenment ideas that gave rise to children's healthcare (James et al. 1998) signified a break with dominant ideas of religious elites that controlled medicine at that time, instead children's healthcare aligned itself with the poor, dispossessed and disenfranchised.

Right from the beginning, the embryonic children's hospitals were formed not in the mainstream established hospitals but in dispensaries or clinics such as George Armstrong's Red Lion Square clinic for the infant poor established in 1769 (British Society for the History of Paediatrics and Child Health 2014). This was more akin to a community health clinic than an inpatient facility; this may explain why children's services have always had more of a community focus.

The founding fathers (*sic*) of children's hospitals were men who were excluded from adult medicine. Charles West founder of Great Ormond Street (1852) was a non-conformist (Lomax 1996), the son of a Church of Scotland minister and therefore not of the 'right' religion to be promoted in the adult hospital. Manchester Children's Hospital was founded by two Jewish brothers (Lomax 1996). Because these men could not or at least felt that they would not be allowed to make progress in the adult healthcare facilities, they created a different space for themselves in founding children's hospitals. In addition to this self-imposed separation, the prevailing conceptions of health at the time also encouraged separate provision. In part due to infamous past failures (General Reception (1756–60) being one), the hygienic movement, of which Florence Nightingale was a key figure, favoured the separation of children on the grounds that children could 'infect' the environment and cause epidemics in the ward (Lomax 1996).

The nurses who worked in these children's hospitals were also seen as being different. In the main, the children's hospitals were funded by charities, with local patrons. These patrons exerted a good deal of influence over the running of the hospitals, for which they were paying, thus the standards demanded of children's nurses were often higher than those expected in other institutions (Lomax 1996). This may have given children's nurses a sense of superiority, which may persist even today!

The association of children's nursing with the fever hospital together with the practices of some hospitals to exclude parents and isolate children may have helped to reinforce the strange otherness of the children's nurse and children's nursing, at least in the public imagination; although arguably in contrast the work of community nurses, including health visitors with mothers and children, has created a more positive image of the nurse. However, again the history both of health visiting and of community children's nursing has been a history of separation. Health visiting did not emerge in the 1890s as a part of adult social work but as a separate health and social welfare service for mothers and children under five (Maxwell 1997; Baldwin 2012) and the history of community children's nursing is quite separate from the development of similar district nursing services for adults (Whitting 2005).

In hospital practice it should be remembered that the call to end the exclusion of parents from the children's ward was not initiated by nurses but by Mother Care for Children in Hospital (1961), which became NAWCH, now Action for Sick Children, a parents' organisation (Action of Sick Children 2013). Nor was it nurses who first highlighted the psychological costs of separating children from their carers in hospital but the James and Joyce Robertson, psycho-analyst and film makers. The isolation of children, and by extension the isolation of children's nursing, was not curtailed by nurses but by social pressures from outside nursing, although some children's nurses have taken up the cause of open visiting and promoted policy to support parents' access.

It seems that nurses have never responded to the social influences of their times with regards to children, nurses did not call for the foundation of children's hospitals in response to the Enlightenment, nurses did not lead the responses to urbanisation and gang cultures which define public policies towards youth in the early twentieth century, nor were the nurses at the forefront of the social changes of the 1950s–1960s when Western culture refocused on the young

(Savage 2008). Although individually many nurses have advocated for many children and young people, the historical record does suggest nurses have something of a blind spot when it comes to shifts in cultures of childhood. This might be characterised as a strong social conservatism, where nurses tend to support traditional professional practices and appear slow to adopt and adapt to changing social circumstance.

Despite the superiority complex arising from the strictures of the voluntary hospitals, the Royal College of Nursing did not have a society for children's nurses until 1984 (Glasper 1995). Children's nursing as a qualification has had a turbulent history and there have been repeated efforts to abolish the specialist qualification (Glasper 2007). Although most countries have some form of post-qualification specialist qualification for children's nursing, and organisations which support children's nurses, many of which are involved in international collaborations (RCN 2014), the UK and Ireland (Irish Government 2010) are the only countries to have programmes in which nurses can qualify as children's nurses as their unique qualification to practice as a nurse. In many countries a double standard exists where children's nurses are not recognised as qualified general nurses but whose skills are much sought after to work in children's areas.

The constant threat that children's nursing will be subsumed into general (adult-focused) nursing, the historical myths of children's nurses as 'superior' and the hard-fought battles over the different requirements that children have as patients, perhaps lead children's nurses sometimes to fight a little too hard: to continue to fight 'for children' even when those around them agree. Being threatened with losing their 'special' status and the undoubted socially disadvantaged positions of children in many cultures (The Marmot Review 2010; UNICEF 2013) arguably makes children's nurses either appear as heroic survivors, battling for the rights of children, or possibly to seem to outsiders as being defensive and protectionist of their role – at times being prone to shroud waving and moral blackmail, laying claim to the moral high ground of 'protecting' or saving children as justification for refusing to critically evaluate professional practices. In either case these are continued residual myths as Arbuckle calls them (2013), myths based on past and now redundant contexts which continue to influence healthcare organisations. For children's nursing, these residual myths would include the belief that children's nurses are unlike other nurses, charged with a special duty to protect children. Such residual myths do nothing to help children's nurses to integrate into the nursing professional group as a whole, but only continue to isolate and separate children's nursing and children's nurses.

In the modern era, children's healthcare was separated from adult healthcare in the main by entrepreneurial men who had their own reasons for founding children's hospitals outside the control of the medical main stream (adult-focused) services. Socially conservative nurses seem to have supported the separation of children and children's healthcare, first by endorsing different standards of training and behaviour for children's nurses, and later by introducing and enforcing the isolation of children from their carers and communities (with the exception of community nurses). These practices which established and enhanced the separation of children in healthcare systems were not challenged by nurses' groups themselves but have in the last 50–60 years been opposed by parent and other professional groups, which some nurses have joined.

Adult-focused theories of children's nursing

Although, as we have seen, the development of children's nursing has taken very different paths from that of nursing more generally (adult nursing), there have nevertheless been attempts to apply theories derived from adult nursing practice to children. The theorising of nursing gained prominence in the 1950s in the main in North America (Meleis 2007). The descriptions of nursing theories often contain a biography of the author, perhaps as a way of linking the theory back to clinical practice. The majority of nursing theorists are nurses who either have a background in acute adult nursing (Benner, Orem) or mental health (King, Roy) and a few are from community nursing (Neuman). Where nurse theorists do have experience of nursing children, they have often chosen not to design theoretical frameworks for children's nursing (e.g., Dorothy Johnson was a children's nurse and professor of paediatrics at the University of California but her theory contains little on children or childhoods (Meleis 2007)).

These general or adult nursing theories share a common assumption which, although not made explicit, underpins each of them. They assume that people exist in a mythical adult state. Like most myths that endure, this 'adult' state has some aspects based in experience, but also some which are fiction. The 'mythical adult' state is a steady state in which no development occurs, it purports to be a frozen moment in the life span. It also seems very often to be a weirdly antisocial state. In the 'adult' state, people have reached maturity, they are cognitively competent and they seem to live independent, individualistic lives with no partners or families. That is, on reading the nursing theories such as Orem or Benner, or even the more psychologically orientated King or Roy, there is little or no mention of how as humans our bodies, minds and relationships change with time as we pass through periods in a life span. Of course in people's lives this 'mythical adult' state never occurs: we all live with changing bodies, and we gain and lose skills and functions throughout our lives. The thymus gland provides a nice example. We are born with a large thymus (in comparison to the rest of the chest organs) which produces naive immune cells ready for exposure to new antigens, but after pubescence to late adulthood the thymus shrinks in size (Askin and Young 2001). There is no point at which the thymus is in a steady state, it changes continuously over the life span.

It may be argued that the fact that nursing theories were designed for adults is less relevant, that they can be adapted for children. Some children's nurses have adapted Orem's self-care model (Burley Moore and Beckwitt 2004), others have used theories of human becoming and caring (Karnick 2005; Lundqvist and Nilstun 2009). Anne MacDonald (1988) describes how she and her colleagues attempted to create a paediatric nursing 'model'. While this Manchester-based project incorporated child development aspects and considered safeguarding, it is based on Roper et al.'s activities of daily living, which were again designed for adults rather than children. For example, the activities of daily living do not address peer relationships or cultures of childhood.

At best these are always adaptations of adult theories. The theories were not designed for children, thus they do not account for many aspects of childhood.

Some nurses may still argue that having a theoretical understanding of nursing is not important. They may claim that they just
do nursing, they do not have to think about it. Unfortunately for
such nurses, this is of course a theory of nursing. O'Toole (2003:
705) defines a theory as:

A basic structure developed to organise a number of concepts
that are focused on a particular set of questions.

Afaf Ibrahim Meleis further defines nursing theory as

a conceptualisation of some aspect of nursing reality commu-
nicated for the purpose of describing phenomena, explaining
relationships between phenomena, predicting consequences, or
prescribing nursing care.

(2007: 37)

The 'natural' argument that nurses just do nursing without thinking
is, in and of itself, a collection of ideas or conceptualisations (often
about women, caring and the instincts of those who chose to be
nurses) which relate to one another (often that caring develops
through experience and cannot be taught) – it is then a theory. What
this brings us to is that there is no atheoretical position on nursing.
As Meleis (2007) points out, nurses may be silent knowers. Based on
the work of Belenky et al., Meleis suggests that some nurses know
their practice and pass their practices on in teaching, but may not
be able to articulate the basis of their understanding or to link their
ideas about nursing to philosophy or other ideas. Meleis does not
suggest these nurses are not nursing, just that their practice remains
hidden and unarticulated. In the case of children's nursing, another
type of 'knower' may also be present: those that are received knowers
(Meleis 2007). These nurses doubt their own and their peers' ability
to generate understanding and instead rely on the expertise of others.
As general or adult nurse theorists have dominated the literature,
in nursing education these received knowers use the understanding
about nursing of such theorists rather than generating their own
understanding about nursing children (Burley Moore and Beckwitt
2004). That children's nurses may not be able to talk about their

practice, have not set it down in journal articles and books (like this one), that they may rely on adult-based theorists is not to say that children's nursing does not exist as a phenomenon about which we can theorise. It simply means that in the past nurses have tended not to do so. As we shall see in Chapter 2 (page 24), pragmatism links our beliefs to our actions, whether or not children's nurses can speak about their beliefs or understanding about children, about nursing they will have such ideas and will act on them. Thus each of us has a constructed theory about the world, even if we cannot put such ideas into words or write books about them. There is no atheoretical position, since to hold such a view on the world, to believe the world is a set of unconnected ideas, would be to have some beliefs about the world which would result in actions and would make a theory (albeit one which stays in one's own head and is only expressed through one's actions).

If we return to adult-focused theories and look at the main constituent of a nursing theory as set out by Fawcett (1995) of person, environment, health and nursing, we can see that each of these pose challenges in relation to applying these theories to children's nursing.

The concept of person is perhaps the most conflicted. The 'adult'-orientated theories consider the person to be the fully cognisant adult who lives an independent life. Children, however, are to a greater or lesser extent dependent on their parents and extended family members as they develop over the period of childhood. Those who adapt nursing theories to be applied to children tend to either suggest reliance on the parents and proxy decision makers or espouse a vague notion of the 'family' being the person.

Important decisions in the child's healthcare may be taken not by them but by others or by proxy decision makers. This is true of adults who are incapacitated by illness, but is not acknowledged in nursing theories, or in many aspects of healthcare. Despite the evidence that children's proxy decision makers' views about how children feel do not match children's own accounts (Noyes 2007) and the methodological arguments advanced by Scott (2008), proxy decision makers are routinely used in children's healthcare within a legal framework of 'best interests'. The concept of 'best interests' is used to frame the decisions taken by one person on behalf of someone unable to make the decision for themselves (see Cornfield and Khan 2012 for a discussion of best interests in practice). While the concept may be a practical necessity, in that there are occasions such as in end of life care where people have to rely on their relatives acting in ways that they think the incapacitated person would want them to act, even the most insightful and organised of us are unlikely to leave sufficiently detailed plans to cover every aspect of healthcare which may be available. As a concept in and of itself, 'best interests' makes very little sense. How can a person tell what would be in the best interests of another person? Even if the outcome of healthcare decisions can be predicted with acceptable levels of accuracy (which is rare), the consequences of one decision in relation to another would rely on the human ability to predict the future. In order to assess what would be in the best interest of the incapacitated individual, the decision maker would not only have to know how likely the medical or nursing intervention was to succeed, but also foretell the effect on the child's life, and would have to do this for a range of possible decisions or actions. This is impossible. The concept is further complicated by the way 'best interests' decisions are supposed to be taken in a non personalised social vacuum, and not be influenced by the person making the decision. It is difficult to be certain that decisions are not influenced by our own preferences, mental maps and cultural understandings, even when dealing with simple unemotive decisions. Many healthcare decisions have such profound effects on the child's carers (parents) and often their siblings and extended family that it is questionable whether an approach which considers in isolation one person's 'best interest' is desirable (see comments below on family-centred care). Consider a family where the second born child has hypoplastic left heart syndrome. Should the parents consent to surgery where the outcome is uncertain and there are risks of further complex health problems (Rempel et al. 2013)? If the family income is low and with the certainty that should the parents consent to surgery the family income is likely to fall as they attend outpatients and deal with long stays in hospital, should the parents put the older sibling's life chances at risk by taking on the care of the sick child? Without the parents' support, the care needs of the child would have to be taken on by the state. This is of course a complex dilemma to which there is no simple answer; however, the 'best interest' of one person, the newborn with a hypoplastic left heart, does not provide an answer.

In trying to understand the person, in nursing theories replacing the child as a person with a vague notion of the 'family' or with a proxy representation of the parent is problematic and unsatisfactory. Yet the personhood of children is also problematic. In many states, children are subject to laws which in effect make them the property of their parents (often their father, see Shields et al. 2003). The United Nations convention on the rights of the child may have widespread (although not universal) acceptance at an official level, yet culturally and often legally children remain the possessions of their parents (Kelly et al. 2012).

For some who have adapted 'adult' nursing theories, the child is a person in their own right, and the family is part of the environment in which the child lives (Lee 2003). This environmental approach at least allows the child to be a person in their own right influenced by the family structures which surround them. What is less clear is the relative influence of the many and varied factors which constitute environmental factors. What is the effect of a difficult relationship with one's mother in relation to lead levels in the atmosphere? The challenge of placing family in the environmental aspect of the nursing theory is how what is a relational factor (Mayall 2008) relates to factors which are physical, such as the chemical composition and distribution of toxins. In 'adult'-focused theories, environment tends to focus on the immediate effects of the environment that the person's body is discovered in, rather than the long-term effects that a toxin or environmental factor might have (the long-term effects of lead for example (Zhang et al. 2013)), or the effects of smoking in pregnancy which affect three generations where the smoking habits of grandmothers affects the health of grandchildren born to the grandmothers' daughters (Hypponen et al. 2003). Nor do adult nursing theories give much attention to the environmental effects on developmental processes; for example, how exposure to background noise affects language acquisition (Pempek et al. 2014) or the effect of using a baby walker has on learning to walk (Ardestani et al. 2008).

While the different conceptualisations of health in nursing theories could be adapted to children's nursing in that health tends to be described in such vaguely universal terms that the concept could be applied to many people in many circumstances (albeit as discussed in Chapter 2 such universalism is perhaps flawed), these ideas do not account for children's developmental processes, or for the social and cultural changes which occur as children progress through their childhoods. It hardly seems reasonable to ignore the effect that developing sexuality and secondary sex characteristics have on people's long-term sexual health and mental well-being, yet such 'adult'-focused nursing theories have no way of accounting for the long-term effects of health decisions taken in the moment which may have long-term effects on health.

Rather like the concept of health, that the ideas about nursing could be adapted to fit children is not the point. Once again the concepts of nursing, like health, are often so universal and nebulous that they could be applied in any situation. But nursing theories designed for 'adults' do not cover how nursing and nurses influence children's childhoods. There is no account of how nurses may at times be called upon to act *in loco parentis*, or of the role of the nurse to support children's carers in their parenting. Despite these aspects of children's nursing being less visible to children and nurses than the support for medical practices (Randall 2010), nurses act every day to directly parent or to support the parenting of children.

'Adult'-focused nursing theories can then be in part adapted for use with children. However, such adaptations face many challenges and ultimately seem to be bound to only give a partial picture of what children's nursing is about. None of the 'adult'-orientated theories accommodate the developmental processes which are so much a part of childhood, with perhaps the exception of Neuman's system model (Neuman and Fawcett 2010) which does feature a life course. However, Neuman's model has not been used extensively with children, nor does it focus on childhood, but rather on a life course more generally. The lack of consideration of developmental processes and of the effects childhood have on children's health make such theoretical nursing models inadequate for use with children.

Lastly there is a moral imperative. Why should children have to receive nursing care which is based on theories and systems which have not been designed specifically for them as children, to reflect their progression through childhood? Why should they be subjected to second-rate adaptations and fudges? Our children deserve better.

Rebuttal of 'family-centred care'

Family-centred care is more of a philosophy of care than a theory. Carter et al. (2014) refer to some attempts to include child and family-centred care as a philosophy or an approach, and while Smith and Coleman (2010) mention theory, they do not set family-centred care within the theory of nursing. Various concept analyses which have been undertaken on family-centred care have failed to find either a consensus on the concept or a coherent theoretical framework (Hutchfield 1999; Mikkelsen and Frederiksen 2011). In general, family-centred care appears to be more a set of values and aspirations about partnership between nurses and parents to encourage parental participation than a set of concepts which relate to nursing and to each other (see O'Toole's 2003 and Meleis' 2007 definitions of theory and nursing theory above). More recently there have been some attempts to recognise children in family-centred care. For example, Smith and Coleman's 2010 second edition of their text has been entitled *Child and Family-Centred Healthcare* rather than just *Family-Centred Care* (Smith et al. 2002). However, the voice of children gets very little attention in the 2010, second edition (most obviously in pages 145–50). The updated text does not consider the agency of children, the sociology of childhood or, to any substantial degree, the role of the state when 'family' care may not be in the child's best interests. Smith and Coleman's (2010) revised book still seems essentially to be about how parental participation can be facilitated and acknowledged, albeit there is an occasional reference to child involvement in care. Nor does the literature on family-centred care answer Fawcett's (1995) criteria for a nursing theory, the concepts of person, environment, health and nursing are not detailed, and it is not explained how they would interact in a proposed 'theory' of family-centred care.

Family-centred care may not be a very well-defined concept (Mikkelsen and Frederiksen 2011), but is, however, a very successful meme. Richard Dawkins (1989) has suggested that ideas can act like genes where the meme (or idea) has an evolution. Memes which satisfy a need and which are sustainable in a community gain strength and evolve, those that do not perish. Family-centred care viewed as a meme has been phenomenally successful. As Smith and Coleman (2010) state, there is hardly a nurse who calls themselves a children's nurse who would not now espouse family-centred care as a central tenet of their practice.

This is in spite the fact that family-centred care is a poorly defined concept which research study after research study has failed to detect in actual practice (Shields et al. 2006, 2007, 2012). Although Smith and Coleman (2010) claim that family-centred care is a socially constructed concept, it seems more accurate to label it a professionally constructed concept. Arguably nurses want family-centred care to exist, but not actually to practise it. Politically possibly they want to be seen as being on the side of parents, but not to relinquish their power to control what happens in the clinical area to parents.

It could be that family-centred care is a useful concept, hence its widespread use, but it's not been well defined, or discovered in practice, not because it is not present, but because researchers have not been looking in the right places or in the right way. It seems highly unlikely but this could be the case, possibly.

Even so, family-centred care seems to have some conceptual flaws. The idea of what a family consist of is ill defined and often politically and culturally contentious. The Institute for Patient and Family Centred Care defines a 'family' as

> two or more persons who are related in any way—biologically, legally, or emotionally. Patients and families define their families.
> (2010)

They go on to state that in the case of children it is parents who define who is in the family, rather than the child. Thus a family by this definition includes anyone that the parent thinks of as a family member. Thus for nurses to truly account for the needs of the family, they would have to account for the needs of a network of people who surround each child, some of whom may rarely see the child, may live in different countries, may not think of themselves as the child's family and may not want anything to do with the child. For many children their family members are likely to come from different generations who may have different ideas on health, childcare and parenting. Increasingly children will have family members who are estranged from their main carers' family, hostility and conflict may still be present and the needs of such fractured families will be complex and often the various factions may have conflicting needs which cannot be reconciled.

Even if children's nurses could wave a magic wand and solve the dilemmas of modern family lives, the effort to do so would, I suggest, leave them no time, energy or resources to meet the needs of the child. Some may suggest that the needs of the child are best served by meeting the needs of the family. However, the needs of the child as an individual and the need to be part of a family are not the same thing. Sometimes the child's needs may coincide with, or be advanced by, conforming to the needs of a family consensus view (if one can be established), sometimes the child's needs will not. The family-centred philosophy allows no consideration of the child's 'best interest' running counter to those of the family.

We need not take the extreme cases of child abuse, where the perpetrators' desires to abuse the child obviously oppose those of the child's welfare (see Southall et al. 2003), but instead consider a more common scenario where the child may require pain relief, but the carer wants to fit in with the hospital culture of not being a 'difficult' parent (Darbyshire 1994). Thus while the child's need is for pain relief, the carer's need is for social acceptance, thus the parent may not ask for the medication and the child suffers, often in silence, as the carer will want to appear to be able to control their child in public by stifling any show of hurt. In this way and so many other small ways, children's needs are undermined, ignored or just overruled by adults.

This is perhaps the greatest problem with family-centred care. It should more properly be called parent-centred care. Its focus is almost entirely on parents, not children – that is, it focuses on the needs of adults as parents not those of children. As is all too often the case, the needs of children are forgotten as adult members of society focus on their own problems (I include myself as guilty of this too). Thus family-centred care, while it professes to be a central tenet of *children's* nursing, is in the main concerned with adults' involvement as nurses and as parents in delivering care, or addressing parents' health and or social problems.

Family-centred care is not just a benign, if rather baggy, concept. It allows nurses to focus on communicating and intervening with parents (adults), rather than taking on the much more difficult and risky task of communicating and intervening with children, with people from another generation. It allows nurses to potentially ignore their duty to stand up for children in an adult world and call loudly for the child's rights often in opposition to the interests of adults, who after all control the societies in which we live. Family-centred care distracts children's nurses and often blinds them to the people they should be caring for – children.

Do we then throw the parent carers out with the bath water? No, as Berry Mayall (2002) has described, childhood is relational – it is dependent on the relationships children have with members of their community, primarily with their main carers. These intergenerational relationships between the child and family members of other generations shape, define and drive the child's childhood. All I am arguing for is that children's nurses focus on children. There are other health and social care professionals expert in helping people sort out their relationships, drug habits or mental health issues. Children's nurses should know what to look for and how to refer on to other services. By all means help parents to parent, but the aim must be to see improvements for the child. Such measures need to be evaluated by the outcomes for children and their childhoods (see Chapter 3).

Earlier in this section I stated that family-centred care is a powerful meme. The power of the idea of family-centred care seems to obliterate the fact that it has not been adequately defined, that it has not been found in extensive empirical research, and that it allows nurses to focus on parents to the detriment of children. It seems likely then that to remove this powerful meme will take more than a few radicals shouting from the sidelines. In part it is hoped that this book might arm a new generation of children's nurses to take up the struggle to refocus children's nursing to be child focused.

Summary

The social construction of children's nursing as separate from adult services in the latter half of the eighteenth century has not been challenged by nurses. The social conservatism amongst nurses, who often support the established status quo, has been challenged instead in the last 50–60 years by parent groups and others from outwith the nursing profession.

This lack of scepticism and critique of children's nursing practice perhaps partly explains why children's nurses failed to theorise children's nursing in the 1950s to 1960s, preferring instead to adapt models of nursing designed for adults. The discussion set out above suggests that such 'adult' models do not account for important aspects of children's development or for their experience of and transition through their childhood.

While the meme of family-centred care has been very successful, spreading widely and helping nurses to secure children's rights in adult-focused health services, it is conceptually flawed. The definition of family is difficult to determine, and the concept does not address where children's interests might lie outside those of the 'family', even if a unified family view could be determined. The danger of using family-centred care to design, deliver and evaluate care is that in repeated research studies no evidence that it is practised could be found. More importantly it seems to allow for nurses to focus on the parents' needs rather than on the child's.

In this book I want to argue that the healthcare of our children should be evidence based and we should understand the cultural, political and social context in which that care is produced, repro-duced, designed, delivered and evaluated. Without such a basis from which to deliver care, children's nursing will continue, as it has in the past, to be subject to social and political agendas, not of children, but of adults.

References

Action for Sick Children (2013) Our history. Retrieved 15 February 2015 from http://actionforsickchildren.org.uk/our-history

Arbuckle GA (2013) *Humanising healthcare reforms*. London: Jessica Kingsley.

Ardestani AT, Honarpishe A and Parsa M (2008) A study on the effect of baby walker on mean age acquisition of motor skills in infants. *Acta Paediatrica*, 97 Supplement 459, 219–20.

Askin DF and Young S (2001) The thymus gland. *Neonatal Network*, 20(8), 7–13.

Baldwin S (2012) Exploring the professional identity of health visitors. *Nursing Times*, 108(25), 12–15.

British Society for the History of Paediatrics and Child Health (2014) 18th century: Dr George Armstrong. Retrieved 15 February 2015 from www.bshpch.com/18th-century.html

Burley Moore J and Beckwitt AE (2004) Children with cancer and their parents: Self-care and dependent-care practices. *Issues in Comprehensive Pediatric Nursing*, 27, 1–17. doi: 10.1080/01460860490279518

Carter B, Bray I, Dickinson A, Edwards M and Ford K (2014) Approaches to nursing children, young people and their families. In Carter B, Bray I, Dickinson A, Edwards M and Ford K (eds) *Child-centred nursing: Promoting critical thinking*. London: Sage.

Cassey A (1988) A partnership with child and family. *Senior Nurse*, 8(4), 8–9.

Cornfield DN and Khan JP (2012) Decisions about life-sustaining measures in children: In whose best interests? *Acta Paediatrica*, 101(4), 333–6. doi:10.1111/j.1651–2227.2011.02531.x

Darbyshire P (1994) *Living with a sick child in hospital the experience of parents and nurses*. London: Chapman and Hall.

Dawkins R (1989) *The selfish gene*, 2nd edn. Oxford: Oxford University Press.

Fawcett J (1995) *Analysis and evaluation of conceptual models of nursing*, 3rd edn. Philadelphia: FA Davis.

Glasper LA (1995) Preserving children's nursing in a climate of genericism. *British Journal of Nursing*, 4(1), 24–5.

Glasper FA (2007) The register under scrutiny again. *Journal of Children's and Young People's Nursing*, 1(4), 157–8.

Howell C (2014) *The Foundling Museum: An introduction*. London: The Foundling Museum.

Hutchfield K (1999) Family-centred care: A concept analysis. *Journal of Advanced Nursing*, 29(5), 1178–87.

Hypponen E, Davey Smith G and Power C (2003) Effects of grandmothers' smoking in pregnancy on birth weight: Intergenerational cohort study. *British Medical Journal*, 327(7420), 898 doi: http://dx.doi.org/10.1136/bmj.327.7420.898

Institute for Patient and Family Centred Care (2010) What is meant by the word 'family'. Retrieved 15 February 2015 from www.ipfcc.org/faq.html

Irish Government (2010) Nurses rules. Statute S.I. No. 689. Dublin: The Stationery Office. Retrieved 17 August 2015 from www.irishstatutebook.ie/pdf/2010/en.si.2010.0689.pdf

James A, Jenk C and Prout A (1998) *Theorizing childhood*. Cambridge: Polity Press.

Karnick PM (2005) Human becoming theory with children. *Nursing Science Quarterly*, 18(3), 221–6.

Kelly M, Jones S, Wilson V and Lewis P (2012) How children's rights are constructed in family-centred care: A review of the literature. *Journal of Child Health Care,* 16(2), 190–205. doi: 10.1177/1367493511426421

Lee P (2003) Children's nursing: Can it justify a separate existence in the UK? *Journal of Clinical Nursing,* 12(5), 762–9.

Lindsay B (2001) Visitors and children's hospitals, 1852–1948: A re-appraisal. *Paediatric Nursing,* 13(4), 20–4.

Lomax E (1996) *Small and special: The development of hospitals for children in Victorian Britain.* London: Welcome Institute for the History of Medicine.

Lundqvist A and Nilstun T (2009) Noddings caring ethics theory applied in a paediatric setting. *Nursing Philosophy,* 10(2), 113–23.

MacDonald A (1988) A model for children's nursing. *Nursing Times,* 84(34), 52–5.

The Marmot Review (2010) *Fair society, healthier lives: Strategic review of health inequalities in England post 2010.* London: The Marmot Review.

Maxwell J (1997) Children and state intervention: Developing a coherent historical perspective. In Rafferty AM, Robinson J and Elkan R (eds) *Nursing history and the politics of welfare.* London: Routledge.

Mayall B (2002) *Towards a sociology for childhood: Thinking from children's lives.* Birmingham: Open University Press.

Mayall B (2008) Conversations with children: Working with generational issues. In Christensen P and James A *Research with children: Perspectives and practices,* 2nd edn (pp. 109–25). Abingdon: Routledge.

Meleis AI (2007) *Theoretical nursing: Development and progress,* 4th edn. Philadelphia: Lippincott Williams & Wilkins.

Mikkelsen G and Frederiksen K (2011) Family-centred care of children in hospital – a concept analysis. *Journal of Advanced Nursing,* 67(5), 1152–62. doi: 10.1111/j.1365–2648.2010.05574

Neuman B and Fawcett J (eds) (2010) *The Neuman systems model,* 5th edn. Upper Saddle River, NJ: Pearson.

Noyes J (2007) Comparison of ventilator-dependent child reports of health related quality of life with parent reports and normative populations. *Journal of Advanced Nursing,* 58(1), 1–10. doi: 10.1111/j.1365–2648.2006.04191.x

O'Toole MT (2003) *Millar-keane encyclopedia, dictionary of medicine, nursing and allied health,* 7th edn. Philadelphia: Saunders.

Pempek TA, Kirkorian HL and Anderson DR (2014) The effects of background television on the quantity and quality of child-directed speech by parents. *Journal of Children and Media,* 8(3), 211–22. doi: 10.1080/17482798.2014.920715

Randall D (2010) *'They just do my dressings': Children's perspectives on community children's nursing.* Unpublished PhD thesis, University of Warwick, Warwick.

Rempel GR, Ravindran V, Rogers LG and Magill-Evans J (2013) Parenting under pressure: A grounded theory of parenting young children with lifethreatening congenital heart disease. *Journal of Advanced Nursing,* 69(3), 619–30. doi: 10.1111/j.1365–2648.2012.06044.x

Royal College of Nursing Adolescent Health Forum (2008) *Adolescence: Boundaries and connections: An RCN guide.* London: Royal College of Nursing.

Royal College of Nursing Children and Young People's Mental Health Forum (2008) *Lost in transition: Moving young people between child and adult health services.* London: Royal College of Nursing.

Royal College of Nursing (2014) International Association of Paediatric Nurses. Retrieved 15 February 2015 from www.rcn.org.uk/development/communities/rcn_forum_communities/children_and_young_people_field_of_practice/other_forums_and_groups/international_association_of_paediatric_nurses

Savage, J (2008) *Teenage: The creation of youth 1875–1945*. London: Pimlico.

Scott, J (2008) Children as respondents: The challenge for quantitative methods. In Christensen P and James A (eds) *Research with children: Perspectives and practices*, 2nd edn (pp. 87–109). Abingdon: Routledge.

Shields L, Kristensson-Hallstrom I, Krisjansdottir G and Hunter J (2003) Who owns the child in hospital? A preliminary discussion. *Journal of Advanced Nursing*, 41(3), 213–22.

Shields L, Pratt J and Hunter J (2006) Family centred care: A review of qualitative studies. *Journal of Clinical Nursing*, 15(6), 1317–23.

Shields L, Pratt J, Davis L and Hunter J (2007) Family-centred care for children in hospital. *Cochrane Database Systematic Reviews* 2007 (CD004811). doi: 10.1002/14651858.CD004811.pub2

Shields L, Zhou H, Pratt J, Taylor M, Hunter J and Pascoe E (2012) Family-centred care for hospitalised children aged 0–12 years. *Cochrane Database of Systematic Reviews*, 10 (CD004811). doi: 10.1002/14651858.CD004811.pub3.

Southall DP, Samuels MP and Golden MH (2003) Classification of child abuse by motive and degree rather than type of injury. *Archives of Disease in Childhood*, 88(2), 101–4.

Smith L and Coleman V (eds) (2010) *Child and family-centred healthcare: concept, theory and practice*, 2nd edn. Basingstoke: Palgrave Macmillan.

Smith L, Coleman V and Bradshaw M (eds) (2002) *Family centred care: Concepts, theory and practice*. Basingstoke: Palgrave.

UNICEF (2013) The state of the world's children 2013: Children with disabilities. New York: United Nations Children's Fund (UNICEF). Retrieved 17 August 2015 from www.unicef.org/sowc2013/files/SWCR2013_ENG_Lo_res_24_Apr_2013.pdf

Whitting M (2005) 1888–2004: A historical overview of Community Children's Nursing. In Sidey A and Widdas D (eds) *Textbook of community children's nursing*, 2nd edn (pp. 17–41). Edinburgh: Elsevier.

Williams AN (2007) Four candles. Original perspectives and insights into 18th century hospital child healthcare. *Archives of Disease in Childhood*, 92, 75–9. doi: 10.1136/adc.2006.095729.

Zhang N, Baker HW, Tufts M, Raymond RE, Salihu H and Elliott MR (2013) Early childhood lead exposure and academic achievement: Evidence from Detroit public schools, 2008–2010. *American Journal of Public Health*, 103(3), e72–e77. doi: 10.2105/AJPH.2012.301164

2 Assumptions about understanding, nursing, children and childhoods

Introduction

The label of pragmatist is often used to refer, in a less than flattering light, to someone who ignores principles in favour of any means which allow them to achieve their goals. In this book, pragmatism is explored as a theoretical framework, which informs our understanding of children's nursing. I will set out the ideas of pragmatism that have developed from its origins in the Metaphysical Club in mid-nineteenth-century America to twenty-first-century perspectives. I argue that pragmatism has particular features which mean it works well with ideas about childhood. Ideas about both pragmatism and childhood rely on the context in which they occur. They both relate to the time in which they occur; in other words, they are temporal. Both sets of ideas also relate to where they occur and to the spaces they occupy, which is physical and geographical but also political and cultural. Pragmatism and childhood can then be situated in time and space, and I argue so can children's nursing. Pragmatism locates children's nursing within political, cultural and social landscapes of its time, and within a story of the history, and current circumstance of humans.

A pragmatic approach offers children's nurses a way to account for the phenomena of children's nursing and to understand how children's nursing helps children to live a childhood where they also live with illness and or life-limiting/threatening disease at a particular time in their communities.

Pragmatism

The Metaphysical Club at Harvard, Massachusetts, USA in 1871 was the crucible in which pragmatism was forged primarily by Charles Peirce and William James, inspired by the ideas of Alexander Bain. The book by John P Murphy (1990) gives an excellent introduction to pragmatism and charts its development from the late nineteenth century to modern figures such as Davidson and Rorty. I shall not attempt here to reprise the entire history of pragmatism, but merely to apply the concepts of pragmatism to the practice of children's nursing. As Richard Rorty (1999) has pointed out, the time for pragmatism may be upon us. Pragmatism was formed at a time of change in the world of science; Peirce was influenced by Darwin's revolutionary thesis in 1860. Similarly Dewey, then Quine, Davidson and Rorty were writing at a time when the 'fundamentals' of understanding about science and reality were being contended by postmodernism. Pragmatism is perhaps, at least in part, a reaction to the shifting sands of understanding that is evident in a post-structural/postmodern society. James' phrase could be a mantra for these times of change:

> We have to live today by what truth we can get, and be ready tomorrow to call it falsehood.
>
> (Murphy 1990: 50)

Based on the discussion in Chapter 1, we might argue that where previously children's nurses held that ill children are best separated from their parents, this is no longer a view that is supported. Thus, just as James said, what we once held to be true is now seen as false. Bearing James' mantra in mind, I want to look at the principles of pragmatism and what they might mean for children's nursing.

Peircian pragmatism links belief and action. For Peirce, thought is brought about by doubt. A nurse would have doubts about how children should be treated in healthcare. Should they be a possession of their parents, a subject of parental rights? Or are they independent individuals with their own needs, wishes and desires? Doubts about such matters would, according to Peirce's view, drive nurses' thoughts. The state of doubt is uncomfortable, it irritates, such that the nurse will be moved to resolve the doubt into a belief, or a more settled view which they are able to accommodate and which relieves the feeling of irritating doubt. Perhaps the nurse moves to the belief that children are individuals, and parental rights are a social construction. Such a belief would show itself in a set of actions, these in turn would give rise to more doubt – for example, how should nurses interact with preverbal children? Thought arises from doubt and seeks relief in belief, belief results in actions, actions in turn raise more doubts (Figure 2.1).

Peirce held that belief and actions define phenomena. Thus there is no aspect of children's nursing which is not accounted for by the actions which reflect people's belief about children's nursing. Further Peirce stated:

> Consider what effects, that might conceivably have practical bearing, we conceive the object of our conception to have. Then our conception of these effects is the whole of our conception of the object.
>
> (Murphy 1990: 27)

Thus if our conception or beliefs about children's nursing have no observable effects, then they are not about children's nursing. Shields

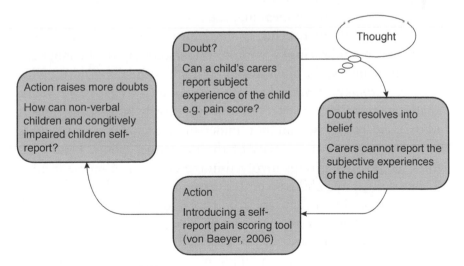

Figure 2.1 Pragmatic children's nursing

et al. (2007, 2012) have shown in their Cochrane reviews of family-centred care that there is very poor evidence that nurses demonstrate family-centred care, thus if adopting a pragmatic approach we have to question if family-centred care is a part of children's nursing (see Chapter 1, p. 14).

Pragmatism only permits 'sensible' questions to be asked. While one could ask all sorts of questions about children, and about nursing, Peircian pragmatism requirements of belief and action and consideration of the effect of action prompts us to ask questions which will have implications for the actions we are to take in the practice of children's nursing. Thus the only questions worth asking are ones which will have implications for the actions which in turn will define children's nursing. A pragmatic approach then to children's nursing would consider which questions will result in actions that will effect children's nursing.

Dewey then Quine considered the role of language and meaning or belief in Peircian terms. Pragmatists refute the idea that language is a labelling system akin to that which might be used in a museum, where a change of language would simply entail changing the labels on the exhibits (Murphy 1990: 80). Instead, Dewey proposed that meaning and behaviour (or in Peircian terms, belief and action) are linked as interactions of at least two people who belong to an organised group with its own habits of speech. Quine expanded on the relationship between meaning, intention and behaviour. He uses the analogy of an alien being beamed into a children's ward (well alright I am paraphrasing) – with no understanding of the language of children's nurses, the alien would be stuck with what Quine called *the indeterminacy of radical translation* (Murphy 1990: 84). While the alien may be able to determine which words label some objects and/or concepts, it would not understand the meaning of these labels, because it is not a part of the organised group. Figure 2.2 details the possible groups involved in the child–carer–nurse triad.

If one substitutes child or indeed carer for alien, there is a clear danger that children's nurses could develop meanings to which children and their carers may not be party. Arguably this is the problem of family-centred care developed as a 'professional' concept understood in the language of children's nurses, but not by children or their carers and families. A pragmatic approach to children's nursing must be mindful of the communities included in the practice and the potential for ideas about the profession to exclude people from understanding and practices of children's nursing (see Chapter 5).

This focus on the practical implication may seem obvious when considering a practice such as children's nursing. However, Murphy (1990) suggests that Peircian 'effects' should include consideration of all possible effects. If 'sensible' questions are to consider all possibilities which may have effects on children's nursing, consideration has also be given to the values and to the political, ethical and legal principles which underpin the practice of nursing children.

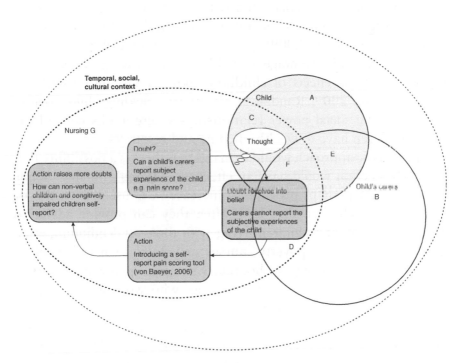

A Child understanding does not match carers nor nurses e.g. peer cultures

B Carers' understanding does not match child's nor nurses e.g. adult agendas

C The child and nurse share understanding but carers do not e.g. supported self-management

D The carer and nurse share understanding, but the child does not e.g. therapeutic holding

E Carer and child share understanding, but the nurse does not e.g. family history

F Child, carer and nurse share understanding (ideal state)

G Nurse understanding not shared with child nor carers (much of nursing literature and professional agendas)

Figure 2.2 Communities and cultures of children's nursing

Children's nursing is a moral practice, in that children's nursing aims to 'do good' (see further discussion in Chapter 5).

Perhaps an example would be helpful here to give some more concrete shape to the argument. We could consider whether nurses should address child poverty. Poverty has an impact on children's health (The Marmot Review 2010; Randall et al. 2010), thus it could be reasonable to consider the nurse's role in tackling poverty. Is the nurse role in child poverty a 'sensible' inquiry?

Certainly the evidence that poverty affects the health of children raises doubt about the role of the nurse (The Marmot Review 2010). If we accept that nursing is not just the restoration of function, but also the promotion of health and well-being (RCN 2014), then nurses are surely concerned with children's poverty. Living in poverty affects children's mental and physical health (Yoos et al. 2009; Melchior et al. 2009). Child poverty puts children not only in a position of disadvantage as children, but growing evidence also suggests that the effects of childhood poverty last into adulthood (Kendall et al. 2009; Randall et al. 2010). Tackling child poverty challenges the social power relationships where adults control the access children have to wealth, income and resources.

A pragmatic approach would demand that there is a possibility that the nurse's action would have an effect on children's nursing. While nurses cannot perhaps provide an increase in household wealth or income to all children they look after, they can provide advice to parents looking after children living with illness (Glendinning et al. 2001). In relation to poverty, nurses may fulfil Joan Liaschenko's (1997) vision of nursing as a boundary subject, signposting carers of children to other resources and agencies who work with clients to increase their income and maximise the use of resources.

Thus the nurse's role in addressing child poverty is a 'sensible' inquiry by the criteria set out above for pragmatism. The resolution of this doubt of course leads to belief which is seen in action. Some nurses do indeed advise carers of children how to access local and national resources such as education, welfare benefits and financial advice (Abbott and Hobby 2003). For health visiting colleagues, such actions are a part of routine practice (DH 2011). The action is underpinned by a belief that children should be able to have fair access to the resources of their society, that societies need to invest in their children as children and as future adult citizens, and that such investment pays dividends in terms of children's health and later their health as adults (Kendal et al. 2009).

Murphy sums up Peircian pragmatism's view of truth thus:

> What is true in our way of thinking is the production of beliefs that prove themselves to be good, and good for definite assignable reasons.
>
> (1990: 57)

We will return to the arguments of what is good and good for whom in Chapter 5. For now, the resolution of the doubts about the nurse's role in child poverty into a set of beliefs about nursing, child poverty and the interaction of nurses and parents (as set out above) also leads, as Peirce predicted, to more doubt. For example: how best can nurses advise carers? What is the role of the nurse where resources are being diverted to meet adults' needs at the expense of children? How should nurses interact with the state or other organisations to ensure children living with illness can access resources? And so on.

Time and space

Dewey, who built on the pragmatism of Peirce and James, noted that understanding doubt, belief and action in terms of their effects was a break with the Western tradition of philosophy, a tradition which held that thought related to universal theories. These theories, or philosophies, were derived from an objective Cartesian form, or essence of the thing in itself. Pragmatism, Dewey stated, split from such a view and therefore gives temporal understanding bound by time and space instead of suggesting universal understandings. While universal understandings, because they are derived from the essential nature of a thing, objectively studied, can be applied to all cases in all times and places in all cultures. Temporal understanding, however, applies to certain times and physical/cultural spaces. As Rorty (1982) puts it, all that pragmatism offers us is to understand how things hang together here and now. The temporality of pragmatism means that it is relevant to the time, location and culture in which nurses practise, whereas universalism attempts to force all people, in all

cultures, at all times into a unified theory which is often unsatisfactory. How often in nursing do we say 'one size does not fit all'?

For children's nurses this temporality is helpful, because as James,
Jenks and Prout (1998) have argued childhood is also temporal.
Childhood is temporal because with successive generations it changes
(James et al. 1998). Children's nursing informally already recognises
this. Can one imagine a children's nurse worth anything who does
not know what the current favourites of children's culture are, be
it the Wombles, Harry Potter, Peppa Pig or Frozen? Working with
children is at least in part future focused, as argued below, because
it is in part about preparing children to be adult citizens. Richard
Rorty (1994) has argued that pragmatism is also 'future orientated',
in part due to its modern North American roots.

Just as Dewey argues that the work of pragmatic philosophers
will never be complete as cultures change (Murphy 1990: 77), so
the prospective children's nurse pragmatist will continually have
to test their ideas against a new generation of children living with
illness. An immediate example might be how the internet is changing
self-management of long-term illness not just in the information
available but also the free access young people who are growing up
with the internet are demanding (Chisolm et al. 2011; Corriveau
et al. 2008). The aspect of time and space, in pragmatic children's
nursing, also creates opportunity for nurses to adapt and change
how they practise children's nursing to reflect the organisation in
which they work. Each hospital could have its own version of a
pragmatic children's nursing. The pluralistic nature of pragmatism
would encourage nurses to devise their own nursing practices to suit
the historical development of their organisation and the cultural and
political space in which that organisation exists. We will return to
the political and moral aspects of children's nursing in Chapters 4
and 5, suffice to say here that pragmatists' rejection of the universal
allows nurses to work together in communities to design and deliver
their own pragmatic children's nursing, designed for their communities at that moment in time.

Returning to the question of quick fixes, and perhaps addressing
concerns that such a temporal view of children's nursing opens it to
accusations of being driven by fads and fashions, James answers this
point by offering the following:

Expedient in almost any fashion; and expedient in the long run and on the whole of course, for what meets expediently all experience in sight won't necessarily meet all farther experiences equally satisfactorily.

(Murphy 1990: 55)

Pragmatism is then like a game of chess where one needs to be thinking one, two, three or four or more moves ahead not just about the immediate action of the next move. This has obvious implications for children's nursing. It might seem 'expedient ... in sight' for the nurse to give in to the toddler who refuses to take their medication (because of the immediate sensation of it tasting horrid!) but this in the longer term will not get the antibiotics into the child's system. The lack of antibiotics will in turn allow infection to flourish and that will prevent the child from participating in their childhood. This is just one example of the many ways in which children's nurses have to think through their actions in order to meet care goals in the short, medium and longer terms.

Things are only 'true' as long as they are verified in our experience; if new evidence emerges, we ought to change our belief. Or to put it another way, the 'truths' of today are fallible – to paraphrase James, we have to be ready tomorrow to call our truths falsehoods. Thus pragmatism is temporal, beliefs result in actions within a time and space. James also points to considering how these actions will last over the long term, and that our beliefs and therefore actions may need to be revised as time proceeds and cultures of childhood and of nursing change.

Nursing children

Nursing children is about education in its broadest sense, preparing the next generation to take its place in its society's structure. Enabling transitions through life spans which fulfil socially constructed practices, or as Dewey (1944) states, education is about growing. Dewey argues that life is about change and about growth and that education is how people grow and adapt to their environment, to time and spaces, so to live is to learn and to live is to grow. Education, Dewey states, does not have an end point since to learn prepares people for the next challenge for more learning. Education and here I argue nursing then have value in and of themselves since to receive nursing care is, especially for children, to learn and grow, and to prepare for new health challenges. If an ideal state of wellness were possible, one would still require nursing and learning to maintain the state of wellness in a fluctuating environment and a body which continues to develop and change over the life course.

Not all children globally are able to access formal education; however, it is an aspiration that all children should have access to formal education, and in any case the same argument can be made for children who participate in work as for those participating in formal education (see James et al. 1998: chapter 6) – that is, that children have to live a childhood in order to gain the skills and cultural understandings that will help them live as adults in their communities.

Health promotion is perhaps an obvious aspect of nursing to be suggested as a form of education, containing as it does the concept of health education. Throughout this book I have referred (deliberately) to nursing being for children who live with illness, disability or life-threatening/limiting illness. I have done so because illness and disease often disappear in the literature about healthcare. It is not referred to as the literature on disease or illness, we do not have colleges, faculties or schools of 'diseaseology' but of health sciences or just of health. However, in exploring the assumption about nursing, we need to understand the place of health promotion and education. There is of course a sense in which we all 'live with illness' or at least the threat of illness, even the healthiest of us can find ourselves with a disease or condition which affects our health and/or well-being. Health promotion and education is in a sense disease prevention, or avoidance. Thus all children live with illness; albeit they may not be suffering with a disease or condition at this moment, there is the potential for them to be doing so in the future, or to be recovering from doing so in the past. There is an ever present shadow of illness. This is not the most uplifting of arguments and is perhaps a little limited. There are of course health promotion and education initiatives which maintain children's health status or seek to build their resilience to disease (Avery et al. 2013). The promotion of health and well-being is recognised in definitions of nursing (RCN 2014). What needs to be recognised is that for children the promotion of health and well-being while a part of nursing is also reliant on the participation of a number of other parties. Teachers, social care workers, local authority workers, police, parents, peer groups to mention just a few groups all contribute to children's health. Nursing as an education project certainly plays its part and the pragmatic ideas in this book could be applied to both health promotion and public health work. It is perhaps helpful here to explore further the assumption about nursing being for children living with illness. I think we could and should include in our concept of children living with illness siblings of children affected by disease, disability and life-limiting/threatening conditions. There is a real sense in which these children are also living with the illness, or their siblings' experience of the disease, disability or condition and the experience of other family members of caring for the affected child. Health promotion and education interventions with siblings of affected children would seem to be a part of children's nursing in particular to support these children's mental health (Knecht et al. 2015).

Education is vital not just to the well child or the self-managing child with a long-term condition, but also to the critically ill child. If the internal environment is disturbed, it is difficult to learn. Thus learning is difficult if one's blood pressure is low, one's cardiac system in collapse. Humans prioritise staying alive at that moment not learning for the future (quite rightly, not much point knowing pi if you're dead). Thus the nurse's job is to promote wellness in all children in order that they can learn physical, social and educational skills. For the critically ill child, this means facilitating the practice of medicine such that children return to a state where, with support of their carers (parents, etc.), they are able to learn. The point of highly technical care which might involve close liaison with medical colleagues, or other health professionals, is to return the child to their best functional state.

While nursing is about education, it is not the same as education in the sense of learning to read, write and add up, etc. Learning to read occurs in a social context of children learning alongside other children, or at socially prescribed times, this is children living a childhood. In the case of children's nursing, illness disrupts this process of living a childhood. For nurses to be required, there has to be disease or illness present or at least the risk or threat of disease. The education in children's nursing is set in a context of illness.

Arguably it is the work of parents and other family members to prepare children to enter adult society (see Chapter 3) but it is the work of children's nurses to help children's parents or carers to do this work where disease and illness are present. This may explain some of the negative imagery associated with the children's nurse. Children seem aware of this role of the nurse associated with illness and attach stigma to the child and family who require such assistance, as it is indicative of ill health (Randall 2012).

Adult nursing theories (see Meleis 2007) tend to favour one aspect of health, be it physical (Benner), public health (Neuman) or mental health (King/Peplau), but if children's nurses are to promote this wide sense of education, the theory will have to encompass physical, mental and public/social health. In the pragmatic sense, the children's nursing theory must account for the critically ill child as much as it does for the chronically ill child or the child put at risk by a public health issue. It must encompass physical as well as mental health, because to learn the skills to socialise that are essential to human survival, children must not only be free of physical disturbance to their equilibrium but also be free of overwhelming mental cognitive problems (Feinstein et al. 2006).

Education is not, however, just about achievement, but also about pleasure in freedom, thought and friendships – the essential building blocks of human happiness (see Alain de Botton's (2001) discussion of Epicurus). Education has in and of itself a value as a process, or activity irrespective of the outcome. We can enjoy learning with no exams! Children's nurses need to avoid the view that children are purely beings becoming and ensure that we value children as active participants in the process of learning. As John Dewey stated in *Democracy and Education*:

> Since life means growth, a living creature lives as truly and positively at one stage as at another with the same intrinsic fullness and the same absolute claims.
>
> (1944: 51)

Education is also not a one-way traffic activity: we as adults teaching children learn much about ourselves and our society from helping children to learn. Thus while the outcome of learning, achieving new skills, or understanding are important, so is the process of learning. Being a child in a childhood is as important as living a childhood to become an adult.

The special case of dying?

If children's nursing is about education or growth, in part preparing children for adult life through living a childhood, then how and why would it include care of dying children. Even if we accept that there is merit in the process of 'education' of living a childhood, which may not result in an adult life, the isolation that many children living with life-limiting conditions experience challenges to a degree to which these children are living a childhood as a part of a cohort of children growing up together.

In the pragmatic approach, all aspects of the phenomena need to be represented otherwise they are pragmatically not part of the phenomena under consideration. The literature and the practice of children's nursing certainly give plenty of evidence of palliative and end of life care (Grinyer 2012; Craft and Killen 2007). Thus empirically we should assume that the care of children not expected to reach adulthood is also a part of children's nursing. Models and theories of nursing have traditionally given very little attention to the dying person. Like most medical practice they seem to be more intent on disease and curative focused care, rather than the supportive and symptom focused care, which Bluebond-Langner and colleagues (2007) have suggested is also a feature of palliative and end of life care for children.

As stated above, the sense in which education is being used here is not just about an educational outcome, but also a process. That dying children should have access to this same sense of educational process of living a childhood is not only a moral question to some extent (see Chapter 5, page 95), but also a practical one.

The uncertain nature of palliative and end of life care is well documented (Brook and Hain 2008), so while a child may be expected to die prior to adulthood, they may not. Given that humans find predicting anything difficult, if not impossible (Taleb 2008), it seems sensible to have a dual track or parallel planning approach. One in which children's nurses prepare and guide children through dying (or at least prepare them for the possibility) while also facilitating them living a childhood like that of their peers, as much as is possible.

Even though educational outcomes in terms of traditional educational achievements (GCSEs, A levels or equivalents) or indeed in terms of 'life' skills useful in adult life may not be realistically achieved, the process of education, play, working to achieve skills, receiving feedback in terms of praise, or critique is still of value (Feinstein et al. 2006; Bruner 1977). Again this suggests a parallel planning approach: on the one hand, engaging children in health behaviours aimed at achieving skills and understanding; and on the other, recognising the abilities of children who may have limited functioning, or whose cognitive abilities are being affected by their illness. Balancing the goals of living a childhood as much like that of the child's peers as is possible, and the goals of facilitating a possible death, and managing symptoms may at first seem impossible. Living a childhood and dying may appear to have mutually exclusive goals and actions, but step into any children's hospice, any day of the week, and you will find life being lived in the midst of dying being done.

Summary

The North American pragmatism of scholars such as James, Peirce, Dewey, Donaldson and Rorty offers a way to approach children's nursing which allows children's nurses to understand the time and spaces that children and their carers find themselves in. It means rejecting a universal essential view that we can understand children's nursing as a one size fits all set of solutions which could be applied to all children at all times, anywhere.

The pragmatic approach seems to have some useful synergies with our understanding of childhood. More recent, sociological understanding of childhood suggest it too occurs in a time and space. Using a pragmatic lens to understand children's nursing opens up a new vista of continually changing children's nursing which responds to the cultural spaces in which children live at particular times, in particular places.

References

Abbott S and Hobby L (2003) Who uses welfare benefits advice services in primary care? *Health & Social Care in the Community*, 11(2), 168–74.

Avery G, Johnson T, Cousins M and Hamilton B (2013) The School Wellness Nurse: A model for bridging gaps in school wellness programs. *Pediatric Nursing*, 39(1), 13–17.

von Baeyer CL (2006) Children's self-reports of pain intensity: Scale selection, limitations and interpretation. *Pain Research and Management*, 11(3), 157–62.

Bluebond-Langner M, Belasco JB, Goldman A and Belasco C (2007) Understanding parents' approaches to care and treatment of children with cancer when standard therapy has failed. *Journal of Clinical Oncology*, 25(17), 2414–19.

Brook L and Hain R (2008) Predicting death in children. *Archives of Disease in Childhood*, 93(12), 1067–70. doi: 10.1136/adc.2007.127332

Bruner JS (1977) *The process of education*. Cambridge, MA: Harvard University Press.

Chisolm DJ, Hardin DS, McCoy KS, Johnson LD, McAlearney AS and Gardner W (2011) Health literacy and willingness to use online health information by teens with asthma and diabetes. *Telemedicine and e-health*, 17(9), 676–82. doi: 10.1089/tmj.2011.0037

Corriveau EA, Durso PJ, Kaufman ED, Skipper BJ, Laskaratos LA and Heintzman KB (2008) Effect of Carelink, an internet-based insulin pump monitoring system, on glycemic control in rural and urban children with type 1 Diabetes Mellitus. *Pediatric Diabetes*, 9(Part II), 360–6. doi: 10.1111/j.1399–5448.2007.00363.x

Craft A and Killen S (2007) *Palliative care services for children and young people in England: An independent review for the Secretary of State for Health*. London: Department of Health.

de Botton A (2001) *The consolations of philosophy*. London: Penguin Books.

Department of Health (2011) *Health visitor implementation plan 2011–15: A call to action*. London: Department of Health.

Dewey J (1944) *Democracy and education: An introduction to the philosophy of education*. New York: Free Press/Simon & Schuster Inc.

Feinstein L, Sabates R, Anderson TM, Sorhaindo A and Hammond C (2006) What are the effects of education on health? In *Measuring the effects of education on health and civic engagement: Proceedings of the Copenhagen symposium*, OECD. Retrieved 17 August 2015 from www1.oecd.org/edu/innovation-education/37425753.pdf

Glendinning C, Kirk S, Guliffrida A and Lawton D (2001) Technology dependent children in the community definition, numbers and costs. *Child Care Health and Development*, 27(4), 321–34.

Grinyer A (2012) *Palliative and end of life care for children and young people: Home, hospice and hospital*. Chichester: Wiley-Blackwell.

James A, Jenks C and Prout A (1998) *Theorizing childhood*. Cambridge: Polity Press.

Kendall GE, van Eekelen AM, Li J and Mattes E (2009) Children in harm's way: A global issue as important as climate change. *The Forum on Public Policy.* Retrieved 17 August 2015 from http://forumonpublicpolicy.com/spring09papers/archivespr09/kendall.pdf

Knecht C, Hellmers C and Metzing S (2015) The perspective of siblings of children with chronic illness: A literature review. *Journal of Pediatric Nursing,* 30(1), 102–16. doi: 10.1016/j.pedn.2014.10.010

Liaschenko J (1997) Ethics and the geography of the nurse–patient relationship: Spatial vulnerabilities and gendered space. *Scholarly Inquirery for Nursing Practice,* 11(1), 45–59.

The Marmot Review (2010) *Fair society, healthier lives: Strategic review of health inequalities in England post 2010.* London: The Marmot Review.

Melchior M, Caspi A, Howard LM, Ambler AP, Bolton H, Mountain N and Moffitt TE (2009) Mental health context of food insecurity: A representative cohort of families with young children. *Pediatrics,* 124(4), 564–72.

Meleis AI (2007) *Theoretical nursing: Development and progress,* 4th edn. Philadelphia: Lippincott Williams and Wilkins.

Murphy PJ (1990) *Pragmatism from Peirce to Davidson.* Boulder, CO: West View Press.

Randall D (2012) Children's regard for nurses and nursing: A mosaic of children's views on community nursing. *Journal of Child Health Care,* 16(1), 91–104. doi: 10.1177/1367493511426279

Randall D, Williams R and Wagstaff C (2010) The parent trap: Promoting poor children's mental health. *Poverty. Journal of the Child Poverty Action Group,* 137 (Autumn), 11–15.

Rorty R (1982) Introduction: Pragmatism and philosophy. In Rorty R (ed.) *Consequences of pragmatism* (pp. xiii–xivii). Minneapolis: University of Minnesota Press.

Rorty R (1994) Truth without correspondence to reality. In Rorty R (ed.) *Philosophy and social hope* (pp. 23–46). London: Penguin Books.

Rorty R (1999) *Philosophy and social hope.* London: Penguin Books.

Royal College of Nursing (2014) *Defining nursing.* London: Royal College of Nursing.

Shields L, Pratt J, Davis L and Hunter J (2007) Family-centred care for children inhospital. *Cochrane Database Systematic Reviews,* 2007 (CD004811). doi: 10.1002/14651858.CD004811.pub2

Shields L, Zhou H, Pratt J, Taylor M, Hunter J and Pascoe E (2012) Family-centred care for hospitalised children aged 0–12 years. *Cochrane Database of Systematic Reviews,* 10 (CD004811). doi: 10.1002/14651858.CD004811.pub3

Taleb NN (2008) *The Black Swan: The impact of the highly improbable.* London: Penguin.

Yoos JP, Slack KS and Holl JL (2009) Material hardship and the physical health of school-aged children in low-income households. *American Journal of Public Health,* 99(5), 829–36.

3 Children living a childhood

Introduction

The previous chapter set out the argument for a pragmatic approach; in this chapter I want to explore why nurses need to facilitate children living a childhood. We start by picking up the theme that children's nursing is about education in a broad sense as outlined in the last chapter, then consider why children's nurses should be concerned with facilitating children's childhoods for children who live with illness. Once a childhood focus has been discussed, we move on to consider an educational or growth (Dewey) model of Pragmatic Children's Nursing. We might consider the model to consist of an environmental pre-stage where nurses attend to the internal and external environments which allow, or facilitate, children's access to a childhood. It is difficult to be with your peers and concentrate on a geography lesson if your internal environment is disturbed, perhaps because of low blood sugar. It is also obviously difficult to experience a childhood with your peers if you are isolated in a hospital ward. Arguably once these environmental aspects are addressed (in part if not entirely at any rate), children and nurses can move on to consider who is setting the agenda for the child's care and what the objectives should be. In some degree these aspects are influenced by how such agendas and negotiations are viewed in communities (see Figure 3.1). Alongside thinking about the pragmatic approach, I also suggest eight outcome measures (Boxes 3.1–3.8) which might make useful ways to evaluate practice in a childhood-focused pragmatic way. Finally we need to consider how this pragmatic approach fits with how nurses work in multi-professional teams or interdisciplinary teams. This is of particular importance if we are considering how nurses facilitate children living a childhood as it requires working with other health, social care and education workers equally concerned with children and childhoods.

The purposes or aims of children's nursing

In Chapters 1 and 2 I have mentioned that I think children's nursing is about education and that it should focus on children. What I want to do here is to expand and discuss these ideas in more detail and relate them to children living a childhood.

What I propose is simply that:

> Children's nursing is about facilitating children who live with illness to live a childhood which as far as is possible is similar to that of their peers in their communities.

Why do I think living a childhood is so important? It is perhaps obvious that for children the socially constructed period of their lives termed 'childhood' is of paramount importance. There is of course evidence that the effect of events in childhood influence adult lives and societies (The Marmot Review 2010; Wilkinson and Picket 2009). Recent advances in our understanding of neurobiology are also indicating that events in utero and in very early childhood affect the development of the brain, influencing the person's behaviour for many decades (Kendall et al. 2009). While traditional research on childhood focused on the effects of events in childhood on adult lives, there has now been a great deal of work focusing on children's childhoods as they are being lived (see Prout 2001, 5–16 ESRC programme) and on childhoods in and of themselves rather than just as a pre-stage of adulthood. Our understanding of how children are active social agents in their childhood has also developed in more recent times (James et al. 1998; Corsaro 2011).

As mentioned in Chapter 2, childhoods are temporal, they occur within a particular timeframe, generally accepted to encompass a time from conception or birth to about 18 to 25 years of age (United Nations 1989; Royal College of Nursing 2004). Childhood also occurs in a generational space or context: a cohort of children born around the same time pass through a childhood together and through the rituals of their community on entering adulthood. That Western societies no longer have formal ceremonies does not change the rituals, such as leaving school, passing one's driving test and attending university, which serve as markers of the transition from childhood to adulthood. For many people the children who we grew up with continue to serve as a reference group for our other lifespan transitions (such as forming partnerships and conceiving the next generation). Childhood is not just an individual experience but also one that binds a generation together.

Childhood is important to children in forming their anatomy and physiology, in shaping their behaviour, in providing them with social contacts and in providing them with opportunities to learn. Indeed it is thought that human childhood is so long because of the need to learn complex social, physical and intellectual skills which allow us as humans to survive (Bogin 2006). As stated in Chapter 2, children's nursing can be seen as education in a broad sense. Facilitating children who live with illness to live a childhood is about facilitating them to acquire skills and develop their understanding in order to make connections with their generation as they move through childhood and to prepare them for their adult roles. It bears repeating that we need to consider this education role in a very broad sense as set out in Figure 3.1.

Promote, restore and stabilise health status (internal environment)

For children to learn and to interact with their peers, they need to have a stable health status or internal environment. Malfunctions in human anatomy and physiology tend to present themselves as challenges to our abilities to interact and to function. At a physical and social cultural level, serious illness prevents children from accessing their childhood. It isolates them from their peers, disrupts the relationships which form children's childhoods and affects their cognitive functioning. Thus stabilising and restoring the child's anatomical and physiological functions is a prior step to facilitating other aspects of their childhood. To put it bluntly, there is no point in playing bulldog if you are bleeding out! The aspects of children's nursing which support the practice of medicine often address these internal environment aspects, that is, aspects of children's nursing

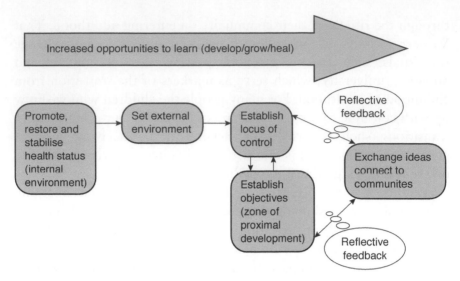

Figure 3.1 The pragmatic education process in children's nursing

that support the interventions and therapies designed by medical and surgical practitioners to restore or stabilise function by addressing the child's physical internal environment. These aspects of children's nursing feature heavily in the literature and in research programmes undertaken by nurses (Glasper and Richardson 2010; Hockenberry and Wilson 2011).

Of course it is not always possible for healthcare professionals to restore health status, or to stabilise anatomical and physiological function. The illness process or trauma may be of such an extent as to mean that the understanding, skills and resources available to the child through the healthcare team are unable to restore or stabilise the child's health status. The child will deteriorate and may die. As discussed in Chapter 2, children's nursing also includes the care of children who are dying and those who live with life-limiting/threatening disease. It is perhaps obvious that promoting a stable internal environment within the child's body is a central plank of dietary and nutritional advice for children. Children's nursing includes reinforcing messages on healthy eating and drinking as well as giving specific nutritional and dietary advice (Howe et al. 2010). In addition, children's nurses care for children who live with disability. Although for these children a stable or restored health status may not be possible, this does not alter the aim of achieving as much function as is possible to allow children to participate in their childhoods. Adaptations may need to be made, participation may be limited or imagined in new ways, but the aim of stabilising or preventing further deterioration in the child's health status to allow them to live a childhood remains the same.

In addition to assessing the physiological health status using paediatric early warning scoring systems (Parshuram et al. 2011), child-focused, health-related quality of life measures could be used to assess the impact of nursing interventions. Existing measures such as the Dartmouth COOP score (Nelson et al. 1990) or PedsQL (Varni and Limbers 2009) could be used, albeit that new measures may be required which provide a validated measure of how such health-related quality of life measures are in turn related to the quality of the child's childhood.

Box 3.1 Outcome measure: health

Extent to which nurses are able to promote, restore and stabilise health status which allows children to participate in their childhood, with their peers in their communities.

Accessing childhood environments

A prerequisite for living a childhood is to optimise physical health status (and by implication mental health status too, being reliant, in part at least, on a physically functioning brain). Learning also requires a stable external environment, we learn best in quiet, reasonably warm environments with plenty of light (Higgins et al. 2005). There is of course a relationship between internal environments or the anatomical/physiological functioning of the body and the external environs in which the body is situated. However, this relationship which is in part physical and in part psychosocial/cultural is not well defined. The nursing literature on the construction of environments is not as plentiful as that on the support for the practice of medicine, but it does exist (Lambert et al. 2014).

In the process set out in Figure 3.1, environment is intended to include the physical and social cultural relationships between the child and their environment, as well as the access to environments in which childhood is enacted. Which is to say, childhood takes place or is lived in a time and a space (see Chapter 2 re pragmatism and time and space). Socially childhoods are assumed to occur in homes, schools, playgroups and communities, whereas illness occurs in hospitals – children know this, which is why they try to avoid hospitals! This is not a new idea in children's nursing, that children should be hospitalised only as a last resort has been extolled as an ideal since the Platt report (Platt 1958). By considering the environment where children live their childhood, nurses can account for children's public health (Blair et al. 2003) and for children's environmental health (Dunn and Burns 2000).

A large part of many children's childhoods are spent in schools. If we include pre-school institutions such as kindergartens (or nursery schools), then even more children and their childhoods would be included. So for children's nurses part of constructing the environment for children's access to a childhood needs to include access to school environments. As noted earlier, while formal education for children, particularly girls, is not universal, it is an almost universal ambition. Nurses should also be very concerned about the working environments that children not able to access formal education may find themselves in (see James et al. 1998: chapter 6). For very many children, and particularly as children move towards adolescence, the school environment is of great importance. Schools provide not only access to formal education, but also a social space for children to socialise with their peers, to enter and withdraw from friendship networks, and to learn social skills. Physical education and sports allow children to develop their bodies and health behaviours, which can influence health beliefs and behaviours into adult life (Department of Education 2013). As noted above, childhood is a cohort activity, and schools give structure to children's progression as a peer group through rituals such as academic years moving from primary education to secondary education or from junior school to senior.

A good way to understand how successful children's nurses are being in facilitating children's childhoods is to look at how much time children spend away from the environments in which their peers are living their childhoods in their communities. This is not just a matter of the percentage of time out of the environment, but also the number of occasions. Part of the effect of being in the childhood environment is the socialisation with peers, the creating of shared memories and experiences which connect children to their peer group. Thus if children are away from these environments, not attending school for example, they are missing these opportunities to create connections with their peers. Particular attention should be paid to ritual events – missing boring history classes is not the same as missing the school production of Oliver Twist (with no disrespect to history buffs). While the hours spent on a subject which a child might not be awfully interested in tend to fade in the memory, other events provide focal points for collective memories of childhood. The outward-bound activity school trip is likely to create memories for children to talk about more than double Maths on a wet Monday.

Box 3.2 *Outcome measure: participating in a childhood*

Numbers of days/occasions children are away from the environments in which they would access their childhood with their peers in their communities; for example, missed school days.

In the education analogy, it may be possible to sit a child in a childhood environment in a kindergarten art room, for them to have a stable internal environment. Their health status may allow them to participate in the art activity, but they do not learn from the experience, they do not develop and change. New skills in social interaction or language do not appear – the child's understanding of social interactions does not change.

Learning requires an objective and a desire or need to acquire the objective. The desire to learn and the objectives of learning are not isolated factors, but are part of a political and cultural context in which ideas are exchanged between members of communities (Bruner 1977). So while restoring and stabilising health status precedes setting the environment and setting the environment precedes the factors influencing the learning objective, the factors of establishing a locus of control (a desire to learn), establishing objectives (deciding what to focus on) and the exchange of ideas form an interactive trilogy each dependent on and influencing the others. To return to my art room example, given that the child in the kindergarten art room has the capacity to learn, they have to want to learn, and to learn identifiable things – to put paint on paper – the resultant blotches on paper are displayed and parents, teachers and/or visitors comment on the child's efforts, other children hear and see these reactions of adults and they too want to put paint on paper. Just sitting in the art room is not enough – one has to interact, to want to paint!

Locus of control

In children's nursing the locus of control, or desire to learn, or perhaps to acquire self-determination, shifts as children mature. For very young children (perhaps for preverbal children 0–2) many aspects of their lives will be controlled and facilitated by their carers and so will many aspects of their healthcare. Although we should consider how children are active in their healthcare even if they are preverbal. Studies in education have indicated how, with imagination, adults can learn a great deal about children's social worlds if adults find ways to communicate with children (Clarke 2005). Young children are of course learning how to move, to ensure their parents feed them and a whole range of skills which are essential for later stages of development. However, for the purposes of children's nursing facilitating a childhood, the point is to recognise that over the duration of childhood there is a negotiation between child, carer (parent) and arguably wider communities, which tends to suggest a move from dependency on carers (parents) towards independence and self-determination, albeit that these concepts are somewhat over-stated in some views of adult cultures. Even if we assume that the child moves from a state of dependence to one of communal membership of a society interdependent on other group members in a community, generally with maturity comes responsibilities not present in childhood. The temporal nature of childhood means that it has a beginning and it has an end, in time (regrettably for us Peter Pans). This shift in the locus of control is of course particularly important in considering how young people transition from children's health services to adult services. With an increasing number of children surviving with long-term health conditions, the issue of transition and this shift from parent-focus care to child/young person self-care has become politically and professionally recognised (DH 2008; Royal College of Nursing 2004).

Box 3.3 Outcome measure: self-care

Nurses can demonstrate how they:

- assess and reassess children's capacity to self-care
- develope children's skills and understanding to facilitate self-care
- encourage and facilitate children to be active partners in their own care.

The general pattern of progression in childhood from dependency to independence as set out above is normally disrupted by illness in childhood. A child who may be starting to assume responsibility for their personal hygiene, for example, may look to their carer to take on the task of washing them again when they are unwell. With illness (or the threat of illness) come nursing needs that make a child and their carers in a sense dependent on the nurse, or at least on the nurse's understanding of nursing care (see Chapter 4). As already implied, children perhaps look to their carer (parents) to meet their nursing needs when they are unwell. However, some health conditions or traumatic changes in health status will require assistance from healthcare professionals. Consider, for example, the child who requires intravenous antibiotics. Parents can and do learn how to administer these; if the child requires them for a chest infection and may require a five to seven day course, it seems to be a waste of resources for parents to learn the skills required and the underpinning understanding of infection control etc. to administer the medication for seven days when the child may never require the treatment again. Even if parents did learn the skills, if the child requires intravenous medication rarely, with perhaps years between episodes, the carers are likely to have forgotten the skills required.

Equally, there seems little point in teaching all parents how to administer intravenous antibiotics if their child may rarely, or never require them. This is the reason we have developed children's nursing as an area of work – to answer the social need in communities for a group of skilled workers who can develop and maintain their skills in providing nursing to children. The example of intravenous antibiotics is a more technical task example, arguably such technical aspects of nursing are increasing with developing technologies. However, we should also consider other aspects where the nurse may be called upon to take a lead. These may be situations where the nurse acts as *in loco parentis*, where for one reason or another the child's own family is unable or unwilling to care for them. This may develop into a situation where the state may formally assume its responsibilities to its young citizens, but more commonly the nurse may act as guidance counsellor and informally resolve situations. It may also include facilitating parental care by allowing parents/carers to take a break, which can help them to continue to care, such as in respite care. A nurse might take the lead where carers need to engage in other activities related to the child's care; for example, providing care while parents discuss care options with the multidisciplinary team, allowing parents to focus on the discussion (whether the child is present for the conversation or not). The ways in which children, their carers and nurses interact is revisited and explored in greater detail in Chapter 4.

In children's nursing, the locus of control will need to be negotiated in tripartite arrangement between the child's own self-care, the care of carers (parents) and the interventions of the nurse. Because the child develops, acquiring new understanding and skills, over the course of their childhood, because during childhood families change and because illness disrupts these patterns, the locus of control in children's nursing has to be continually reviewed and adjustments to care made. Who accepts and who rejects the responsibilities for aspects of the childcare carries with it moral decisions. These moral aspects are discussed further in Chapter 5.

Box 3.4 *Outcome measure: negotiating care*

The nurse has a negotiated plan of responsibilities for aspects of care where the child, their carer and the nurse all have defined and agreed responsibilities in the plan of care. This plan of responsibilities is regularly reviewed and revised.

Objectives of care

Vygotsky's (1962) concept of proximal development may help in understanding how learning objectives relate to children's nursing. In proximal development the learner builds on their current understanding, it is not possible to jump from understanding nothing about children's anatomy to understanding why an infant in respiratory distress needs to be fed small amounts, often. Children's childhoods do not appear overnight: they are the result of accumulated experiences over years. Nor do parents suddenly become proficient at parenting, it takes time, experience and often some blood, sweat and tears! We can say too that children's nurses are not built in a day!

Children's nurses need to be able to locate a child in their childhood and to understand where in the process the child is in order to understand the child's potential for proximal development. They also have to assess the skills and understanding of parents to understand the carer's capacity to parent. In addition, children's nurses have to understand disease and illness as a process.

If we consider Figure 3.2 (which represents a fictitious condition and arbitrary assigned values for health status, purely for illustrative purposes) the parents of each of these children A–C will experience the illness as a continuous stream of events. Child A and their carers/ parents only have their own experience to draw upon, if we discount what they may hear in the waiting room or hospital corridors and parents rooms. And they can only know for certain what has gone before not what may be about to happen in the illness.

A nurse might care for all these children in time periods 1–3. What the nurse can directly experience, which most parents and all children will not, is the process of the illness as experienced by different children over time. Thus in time period 1, the children and

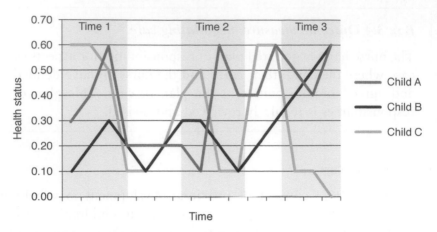

Figure 3.2 Disease and illness process for child/parent and nurses

the parents may despair as the children experience a deterioration of their health. What the nurse can say, from their experience, is that for at least two-thirds of the children things will get better. They can also help children and parents prepare for the possibility of things not improving as in the case of child C. Obviously if the nurse is a reflective and active learner from their experiences, the longer they spend caring for children with particular diseases and conditions the more of this experiential learning they will subsume (Burritt and Steckel 2009). There is then a sense in which nurses too develop via proximal zones. It also follows that nurses will have to keep up to date with medical practice and health service design changes which may affect the child's experience of living their childhood with a particular disease or condition. Thus children's nurses need to understand current research into medical and nursing practices for children and to be able to evaluate the evidence base in order to advise children and their carers on the effectiveness of new treatments and interventions.

If we accept that nurses have a duty of care for children (see discussion below on moral project) such that they ensure, where illness is present, that children receive safe and appropriate care, then they must have the ability to assess the care delivered by family members, most often mothers. Part of setting objectives in care should be setting objectives which facilitate children's carers (mothers) to deliver care. In the main, the motivation of mothers and other carers of children is very high and the nurse may only have to provide some education or equipment in order to facilitate children receiving care from their family member. As discussed above (Chapter 2, p. 34) childhood is relational, it is shaped and formed by the relationships that children have. As Mayall (2002) has pointed out, it is the quality of these relationships that is important, more than with which particular family members they are established. A grandparent or uncle may assume an important relationship to the child providing warmth and a low criticism relationship, even if the child's relationship with their parents is less nurturing. The family member who accompanies the child into hospital or is present in the home may not for that child be the person that they look to for support and comfort at times of challenge such as illness. However, in many cases the main carer who accompanies the child is the person to whom the child looks for such support. Periods of illness can forge and strengthen the relationships for the child and sustain the child and the carer through many years, if not life times, particularly where a child dies. Facilitating care by the child's carer (parents) is not a matter of devolving tasks to save on the nursing budget, but an essential part of facilitating a childhood, as it allows the formation or reformation of relationships which define childhood. It can be argued that, in an ideal world, nurses should be like turkeys voting for Christmas and seek to do themselves out of employment. In utopia, children would be cared for not by professionals but by their parents. For the reasons outlined above, an ideal state is unlikely to occur; nurses will be required, particularly in a technology-orientated world, but one of the main aims of children's nursing should remain to facilitate care by parents (or main carers). It is an important aim because it supports the child in living a childhood.

Box 3.5 Outcome measure: supporting children to live a childhood

Nursing care plan demonstrates understanding of the

• child's position in their childhood

- parents' capacity to meet the child's needs and the skills or understanding that carers/parents need to develop to meet the child's needs
- illness process and how it may affect the child and their childhood.

Where possible the child's main carer feels competent and confident to deliver care and care is delivered by the child's main carer to a proficient standard.

Carers of children tend to be highly motivated; however, motivation alone cannot be enough in some circumstances. Education can be extremely useful and it has been shown on numerous occasions that the more general education a child's carer has the better are health outcomes for the child (Feinstein et al. 2006). Hence the WHO programmes which boost women's education provides great protection for children (WHO 2009). Sometimes what is required is equipment and sometimes the environment in which a child lives requires some adaptation. Facilitating a child's mother (parents/ carers) to deliver care may require a creative and flexible approach (see worked example Chapter 6 pp. 131–7) not mere rule following, but critical and creative thinking. The education programmes which prepare children's nurses need not only to provide the skills and understanding to deliver care, but also develop in nurses the skills, attitudes and understanding to facilitate carers/parents delivering care, which require creative thinking and critical logical reasoning.

Assessment and programmes of developing the child's carers' abilities to deliver care carry with them the possibility that the child's carers may be unable to meet the child's needs, particularly where children have complex care needs and/or server disability. While the majority of parents/carers are motivated to care for their child, some are not. In facilitating the child's carers (mother/parent) to care, nurses also have to be mindful that in order to protect the child or to ensure a reasonable standard of care professional nurses and other health and social care professionals may be required to act. The nurse may be required to take the locus of control away from the child's carer and deliver care themselves, either with some degree of parental carer involvement or exclusively. Children know this to be the case and actively want nurses to stand up for their rights (Randall and Hill 2012).

Box 3.6 Outcome measure: safe care

Nurses ensure the safe delivery of care to children including when appropriate preventing a child's carers from delivering care if it can be established that:

- through the actions of the carer the child is likely to suffer significant avoidable harm
- programmes to facilitate the carer acquiring the required skills, attitudes and understanding have failed.

Nurses act to make appropriate referrals to other health and social care professionals and work with others and carers to develop the carer's capacity to care for the child, either independently or with assistance.

In setting learning goals for carers it may be that other tasks are prerequisites. A carer may not progress, for example, with caring for their child with cystic fibrosis until they have addressed their own alcohol misuse issues. As stated above (pp. 16–17), I do not suggest that addressing these prerequisite issues is the work of children's nurses, just that children's nurses can recognise when a carer is unable/ unwilling to care for their child, and or may need to attend to these prerequisite issues in order to care for the child. They should then make appropriate referrals. Rarely do the circumstances suggest that the carer/parent is to cease all care for their child, normally children's nurses would work alongside other health and social care professionals to facilitate a gradual resumption of the care role as the carer (parent) progresses in addressing the issues. What needs to be clear is that the children's nurses address the development or redevelopment of the carer's care of the child and leaves the work to address the adult carer's problems to other health and social care professionals.

Connecting to communities

The locus of control and the setting of nursing objectives in children's nursing does not occur in a social political vacuum, but rather in communities and at a specified time. Hence, in line with pragmatism, the final element of Figure 3.1 is the exchange of ideas between and within communities. Children's nursing draws on ideas about parenting, about the role of the state in nurturing children, about the agency of children as social actors in their childhoods and about what nursing's function is in modern societies. These ideas are not universal, they are not the same for all children in all spaces at all times, rather they are contextual and pluralistic. There are many childhoods in many communities which change in time and space. Not one fixed formula for all irrespective of time, or where they occur. If we think of recent conflicts and the childhoods for children, the challenges for nurses in Iraq or Syria or Afghanistan are not the same challenges as would have been present even 10–20 years ago in those communities. The challenges which face children's nurses in Australia today are different from those that face nurses in India or Korea (Palliative Care Australia 2010; Partha and Arpita 2013; In Han et al. 2013).

Using a pragmatic approach, one does not demand a prescriptive model that meets all the needs of all children at all times, but rather that the approach accounts for how children's nurses respond to different children living childhoods in different communities at different times. Obviously there are commonalities, a sense in which children are children wherever and whenever they may be.

Box 3.7 Outcome measure: evidence-based care

Nursing care plan draws on current understandings of childhood, parenting, health and social care which are evidence based, with identifiable and accessible sources.

Nursing care reflects the time and space in which children are living their childhoods in their communities, with their peers.

Although using a pragmatic approach should make nurses question such received ideas about children (such as that there is a 'natural' universal childhood), a part of questioning received ideas is to understand how children are viewed in communities. How such perceptions of children and childhood are expressed in legal terms, through case law and statute and how laws are applied in communities affect the rights of children (United Nations 1989). Despite states having different approaches to children and their childhoods, there are processes which allow children's nurses to understand and enact children's nursing, taking account of different circumstances but following principles such as promoting (where possible) care by the child's carer.

Nurses must explore the power relationships which occur as children live their childhoods. The placing of children's nursing in a time and space where different childhoods in different communities are lived at different times requires nurses to consider the cultural safety of the care they offer (Ramsden 2002; Shields and Nixon 2004). As discussed in Chapter 1, children's nursing has often been conservative, in the sense of supporting established elites to maintain a status quo. Because nurse regulation requires nurses to have completed a programme of education, and because these programmes of education are designed, established, delivered and reviewed by elites (established health professionals who claim to have access to understanding not available to all), there is a danger that children's nursing adopts an ethnocentric elite view.

As non-scalable professionalised work (Taleb 2008), nursing may not offer great riches, but it does offer continuous employment at a reasonable rate of recompense (in many countries nurses earn more than the national average and are rarely made redundant (Worldsalaries.org 2008; Robinson et al. 2006)). For a number of interacting factors (such as availability of clinical placements, of mentors and educators), the capacity to educate nurses is often out-stripped by the number applying. Thus educators place barriers to accessing education in order to select the number of applications to match the capacity available. These barriers tend to disadvantage those who come from lower socioeconomic groups, or who are disadvantaged in other ways. Thus the demographic of nursing students tends to reflect the elites of the society it comes from. These students often have the social capital to present themselves as worthy candidates to the educators who control access to the course, they are also more likely to obtain the schooling and educational qualifications that educators demand as entry requirements to nursing courses. There are of course many initiatives designed and implemented to address these challenges, but essentially these are attempts to mitigate for very influential structural social forces and are often limited in their success. The danger then is that children's nurses come from similar cultural backgrounds which are more homogenous than that of the general population. As childhood is a social construction and therefore highly influenced by culture, the lack of diverse cultural experiences or a lack of cultural awareness carries for children's nurses a particular risk. Ethnocentric practice is likely to impose views and conceptions of children, childhood and parenting which can have disastrous effects. Aboriginal and Torres Strait Island peoples in Australia remain wary of health professionals after their experiences of the stolen generation (http://stolengenerationstestimonies.com/index.php/testimonies/index.1.html).

The pragmatic approach with its recognition of different cultural spaces can be useful in reminding children's nurses to be vigilant against cultural imperialism. Children's nurses and nursing needs to ensure cultural safety (Shields 2011; Ramsden 2002) and that children feel the care delivered respects them as individuals from a particular cultural background. Cultural safety is defined by the recipients and is marked by cultural awareness and sensitivity in those delivering care, where diversity and difference in cultural practices are respected (Ramsden 2002).

Among the challenges of putting cultural safety into practice are the dilemmas that cultural relativism can produce, particularly in relation to children and childcare. The late weaning of children on to solid food is an example where the children's nurse may find themselves advocating for a practice – weaning to solid food after six months of breast feeding, which is evidenced based in a Western scientific tradition, but which is opposed by the traditional practices of other cultures, in this case those of South Asian communities (Graham et al. 1997). The views adults have of children and childhood in various cultures make the challenges numerous – ideas on corporal punishment, on the rights of children in decision making, on female genital mutilation to name just a few.

An uncritical acceptance of cultural practice cannot be defended as some cultural practices undermine the other aspects of children's nursing set out above. Cultural practices which undermine the child's rights to expression or which hamper the nurses' attempts to restore health status cannot be tolerated if the critical pragmatic approach set out here is to be taken to nursing children.

Box 3.8 Outcome measure: culturally safe care

The child and their carers feel respected as individuals from a particular cultural background.

Nurses are aware of and sensitive to different cultural practices related to children, childcare and health.

Nurses are able to challenge cultural practice if it can be demonstrated that the practices either adversely affect children's rights in relation to health and healthcare or the practices undermine other aspects of children's nursing interventions.

Nurses may recognise cultural practices and actively seek to modify or eradicate the practice. In the UK, hitting children in the name of reasonable chastisement (*sic*) is permitted. However, nurses can and do suggest that 'smacking' be replaced with positive parenting methods (Wong 2006). Thus a blind acceptance of cultural relativism can be, and is, replaced with advocacy for children's rights in healthcare.

A possible advantage of the approach set out in this section is that it accounts for many aspects of children's nursing which are less visible, acknowledged by children's nurses, often espoused in children's nursing literature, but which have until now perhaps not found a unifying expression. I am thinking here of aspects such as parenting, play, hospital schooling, the provision of social events and outings. These aspects are enacted by nurses every day in the care of children, but rarely feature in nurses' care plans or health service philosophies. They may appear to many as obvious or a natural thing, something we just do – but with a pragmatic approach focused on facilitating children living a childhood, these aspects can be brought together. Providing play facilities and schooling is a part of children accessing the environments which their peers not living with illness would experience, thus the provision of play can be seen as a part of meeting the outcome measure in Box 3.2.

Nursing as a border profession: Joan Liaschenko

The description above of children's nursing has been somewhat simplified for clarity. It may, however, give a false impression that children's nursing occurs between children, their carers and nurses in isolation, whereas nurses are, more often than not, members of a multidisciplinary or interdisciplinary team. To consider how nurses being a part of such teams affects children's nursing, it is useful to consider the work of Joan Liaschenko, who has described nursing as a border subject (Liaschenko 1997; Liaschenko and Peter 2004). Liaschenko's contention is that nursing negotiates and communicates between disciplines or areas of work. The description above can be used to explore this idea in more detail relating to children's nursing.

When nurses are seeking to restore and stabilise health status (internal environment) as detailed above, they are often working between the interests of children, their carers and those of medical practitioners and/or other healthcare professionals. When attempting to facilitate children's access to environments in which to live their childhood along with their peers, nurses work between a number of agencies and institutions and with those who work for these agencies and institutions. The work of nurses here may sit between that of education, housing, town planning, social care, public health and environmental health departments. In relation to the locus of control of care and care objectives, nurses work between the child, their carer and again medical practitioners and other health and social care professionals. When setting care objectives, nurses may also work between the interests of the child and those of researchers seeking to advance understanding on children's health or commissioners evaluating the use of resources in children's health services. When addressing the exchange of ideas in communities, nurses may again find themselves discussing the concepts with other education, health and social care workers, researchers and with policy makers.

Standing in the position between all these areas of interest holds for nurses and for children's nursing some potential vulnerability. Liaschenko (1997) uses the analogy of healthcare as a landscape where the view of the land is synonymous with power and by association with funding and the allocation of other resources in healthcare. Often Liaschenko suggests the practice of medicine sits as a very large mountain in the foreground blotting out other aspects of healthcare which are there, but are hidden behind the bulk of medical practice. Being less visible and therefore given less attention, afforded less power and therefore less resources, including financial support, makes the hidden aspects vulnerable. Because the work of nurses with children does not lay claim to a unique body of knowledge or position in the healthcare landscape, it is often less visible than work which can be attributed to a single professional group (who often lobby those who allocate resources on the importance of their own particular professional group). Thus the border work which is required to facilitate children living their childhood is particularly invisible.

This spatial vulnerability, as Liaschenko terms it, has practical implications with associated costs and challenges (Randall 2010). Nurses understand and value the work between agencies and professional groups to facilitate children's childhoods, but it may not be recognised or often rewarded in the healthcare system. Many nurses dedicate time, energy and creativity to undertake this border work, however, they are also healthcare professionals and they have to attend to the aspects which the funders and managers of healthcare see as important. The workload for nurse is then increased, with the less visible undervalued but essential work being added to more visible tasks valued by healthcare management. Containing such a burdensome workload within contracted hours is often difficult, thus many nurses pay the cost for undertaking the less visible border work by working extended hours. This reduces the time and energy they can spend on their own social lives, including family lives, which in turn has a cost in terms of the nurse's mental health. Long working hours and heavy workloads are contributing factors to nursing's high 'burn out' rates (Sawbridge and Hewison 2013). Those that refuse to sacrifice their personal time and energy in this way are likely to be sanctioned, often by their work colleagues socially isolating them and by managers giving promotions or other opportunities (such as study leave/funding) to staff who are seen as 'team players', that is, who sacrifice their own time to meet the dual requirements of visible and less visible work.

If the less visible border work which allows children to live their childhood is recognised by funders and managers, it often remains at the margins of the work nurses do. The less visible work is vulnerable to being lost when resources are scarce or when the demand to focus on the more visible practice of medicine increases. Aspects of children's nursing such as liaison work with schools providing play or facilitating children access to social events are often seen by managers and funders as 'nice optional extras' or part of an unaffordable gold standard service, whereas the pragmatic approach focused on children's childhoods outlined here suggest these are vital aspects of nurses' work in facilitating the child's childhood.

Part of the point of writing this book is to make the work of nurses in children's childhoods more visible in the hope that by making the work visible it can move to the centre ground in the healthcare landscape and become less marginalised, more secure in its resourcing and less vulnerable to being overlooked and lost.

Summary

By refocusing children's nursing on how nurses facilitate children who live with illness, disability or life-limiting/threatening disease to live a childhood, we can see that children's nursing as a process is similar to learning. By using the framework of a learning model, we have explored the aims of children's nursing.

Children's nursing requires two prerequisites: first, the restoration and stabilising of the internal environment or health status; second, the arrangement of the environment to enhance health status and allow access to childhood environments. With these in place, or at least with plans to address them in place, the nurse can set out a plan of care which allocates roles and responsibilities to the child, to themselves as nurses and to the child's carers. The plan should be based on an understanding of the child's childhood, on the capacity for self-care of the child and of the child's carers' capacity to deliver care, with an aim to increase the skills and understanding of both children and their carers, and the child managing their own healthcare, where possible. The pragmatic approach set out here demands that nurses explore the power relationships between all those involved in delivering nursing care, recognising that children will live different childhoods in different times in communities which may differ. Such a reflexive understanding does not allow nurses just to observe and not act – as in pragmatism, belief results in action. Thus while nurses may value difference, they are also required to act to safeguard children's rights and to ensure children receive safe and appropriate care by making the aim of children's nursing to

> facilitate children who live with illness to live a childhood, which as far as is possible is similar to that of their peers, in their communities.

Many of the aspects of children's nursing which nurses recognise and value, but which people who control the resources in healthcare may not value, become more visible and assume their proper importance. Aspects such as providing play, which has been marginalised in healthcare, can be seen as a vital part of children accessing childhood environments, as opportunities for children to be with their peers and to construct shared memories which bind a generation of children to each other and to their childhoods, that play is integral to the time and space in which children's childhoods occur. That playing together establishes and re-establishes the relationships which are integral to the child's experience of childhood.

The approach taken is pragmatic in that it attempts to account for all aspects of the phenomena of children's nursing; drawing on published literature, it does not rely on a universal unified view but recognises the time and space in which children's nursing occurs and values the differences between cultures of childhood. The approach is also critical in that it demands that the received ideas about children's nursing and the power relationship upon which these are based are explored and challenged. The relationships which frame and contain children's nursing is the subject of the next chapter.

References

Blair M, Stewart-Brown S, Waterston T and Crowther R (2003) *Child public health*. Oxford: Oxford University Press.

Bogin B (2006) Modern human life history: The evolution of human childhood and fertility. In Hawkes K and Paine RR (eds) *The Evolution of human life history* (pp. 197–230). Santa Fe, NM: School of American Research Press.

Bruner JS (1977) *The process of education*. Cambridge, MA: Harvard University Press.

Burritt J and Steckel C (2009) Supporting the learning curve for contemporary nursing practice. *Journal of Nursing Administration*, 39(11), 479–84.

Clark A (2005) Ways of seeing using the Mosaic approach to listen to young children's perspectives. In Clark A, Trine Kjorholt A and Moss P (eds) *Beyond listening children's perspectives on early child hood services* (pp. 29–51). Bristol: Policy Press.

Corsaro WA (2011) *The sociology of childhood*, 3rd edn. Thousand Oaks, CA: Pine Forge Press/Sage.

Department of Education (2013) *Evidence on physical education and sport in schools: Key findings*. London: Department of Education. Retrieved 17 August 2015 from www.gov.uk/government/uploads/system/uploads/attachment_data/file/226506/Evidence_on_physical_education_and_sport_in_schools-summary.pdf

Department of Health (2008) *Transition: Moving on well. A good practice guide for health professionals and their partners on transition planning for young people with complex health needs or a disability*. London: Department of Health.

Dunn AM and Burns CE (2000) Environmental health. In Burns CE, Brady MA, Dunn AM and Starr NB (eds) *Pediatric primary care: A handbook for nurse practitioners*, 2nd edn (pp. 1281–309). Philadelphia: WB Saunders.

Feinstein L, Sabates R, Anderson TM, Sorhaindo A and Hammond C (2006) What are the effects of education on health? In OECD, *Measuring the effects of education on health and civic engagement: Proceedings of the Copenhagen symposium*, OECD. Retrieved 17 Ausust 2015 from www1.oecd.org/edu/innovation-education/37425753.pdf

Glasper EA and Richardson J (eds) (2010) *A textbook of children's and young people's nursing*, 2nd edn. Edinburgh: Churchill Livingston/ Elsevier.

Graham EA, Carlson TH, Sodergren KK, Detter JC and Labbe RF (1997) Delayed bottle weaning and iron deficiency in Southeast Asian toddlers. *Western Journal of Medicine*, 167(1), 10–14.

Higgins S, Hall E, Wall K, Woolner P and McCaughey C (2005) *The impact of school environments: A literature review*. Newcastle upon Tyne: Design Council and University of Newcastle.

Hockenberry MJ and Wilson D (eds) (2011) *Wong's nursing care of infants and children (multimedia enhanced version)*. St Louis: Mosby/Elsevier.

Howe R, Forbes D and Baker C (2010) Providing optimum nutrition and hydration. In Glasper AE, Aylott M and Battick C (eds) *Developing practical skills for nursing children and young people* (pp. 203–28). London: Hodder Arnold.

In Han S, Sang AK and Woong-Sub P (2013) Family factors associated with children's handwashing hygiene behavior. *Journal of Child Health Care*, 17(2), 164–73. doi:10.1177/1367493512456106

James A, Jenks C and Prout A (1998) *Theorizing childhood*. Cambridge: Polity Press.

Kendall GE, van Eekelen AM, Li J and Mattes E (2009) Children in harm's way: A global issue as important as climate change. *The Forum on Public Policy*. Retrieved 17 August 2015 from http://forumonpublicpolicy.com/spring09papers/archivespr09/kendall.pdf

Lambert V, Coad J, Hicks P and Glacken M (2014) Young children's perspectives of ideal physical design features for hospital-built environments. *Journal of Child Health Care*, 18(1), 57–71. doi: 10.1177/1367493512473852

Liaschenko J (1997) Ethics and the geography of the nurse–patient relationship: Spatial vulnerabilities and gendered space. *Scholarly Inquiry for Nursing Practice*, 11(1), 45–59.

Liaschenko J and Peter E (2004) Nursing ethics and conceptualisations of nursing: Profession, practice and work. *Journal of Advanced Nursing*, 46(5), 488–95.

The Marmot Review (2010) *Fair society, healthier lives: Strategic review of health inequalities in England post 2010*. London: The Marmot Review.

Mayall B (2002) *Towards a sociology for childhood: Thinking from children's lives*. Birmingham: Open University Press.

Nelson EC, Landgraf JM, Hay RD, Wasson JH and Kirk JW (1990) The functional status of patients: How can it be measured in physicians offices. *Medical Care*, 28(12), 1111–26.

Palliative Care Australia (2010) *Journeys: Palliative care for children and teenagers*, 2nd edn. Canberra: Commonwealth of Australia.

Parshuram CS, Duncan HP, Joffe AR, Farrell CA, Lacroix JR, Middaugh KL, Hutchison JS, Wensley D, Blanchard N, Beyene J and Parkin PC (2011) Multicentre validation of the bedside paediatric early warning system score: A severity of illness score to detect evolving critical illness in hospitalised children. *Critical Care*, 15(4), R184 doi: 10.1186/cc10337

Partha D and Arpita D (2013) Inequality in child mortality across different states of India: A comparative study. *Journal of Child Health Care*, 17(4), 397–409. doi: 10.1177/1367493512468359

Platt H (1958) *The welfare of children in hospital*. London: Central Health Services, HMSO.

Prout A (2001) Representing children: Reflections on the children 5–16 programme. *Children and Society*, 15(3), 193–201. doi: 10.1002/chi.667

Ramsden I (2002) Cultural safety and nursing education in Aotearoa and Te Waipounamu. Retrieved 17 August 2015 from http://www.nzno.org.nz/Portals/0/Documents/Services/Library/2002%20RAMSDEN%20I%20Cultural%20Safety_Full.pdf

Randall D (2010) 'They just do my dressings': Children's perspectives on community children's nursing. Unpublished PhD thesis, University of Warwick, Warwick.

Randall D and Hill A (2012) Consulting children and young people on what makes a good nurse. *Nursing Children and Young People*, 24(3), 14–19.

Robinson S, Cox S and Murrells T (2006) Developing the children's nursing workforce: Profile, first jobs and future plans of newly qualified diplomats. *Journal of Child Health Care*, 10(1), 55–68. doi: 10.1177/1367493506060207

Royal College of Nursing (2004) *Adolescent transition care: Guidance for nursing staff*. London: Royal College of Nursing.

Sawbridge Y and Hewison A (2013) Thinking about the emotional labour of nursing – supporting nurses to care. *Journal of Health Organization and Management*, 27(1), 127–33. doi: 10.1108/14777261311311834

Shields L (2011) Family centred care: Effective care delivery or sacred cow? *Forum on Public Policy*. Retrieved 17 August 2015 from forumonpublicpolicy.com/vol2011.no1/archive2011.no1/shields.pdf

Shields L and Nixon J (2004) Hospital care of children in four countries. *Journal Advanced Nursing*, 45(5), 475–86.

Taleb NN (2008) *The Black Swan: The impact of the highly improbable*. London: Penguin.

United Nations (1989) *Convention on the rights of the child*. Geneva: United Nations.

Varni JW and Limbers CA (2009) The pediatric quality of life inventory: Measuring pediatric health-related quality of life from the perspective of children and their parents. *Pediatric. Clinics of North America*, 56(4), 843–63. doi: 10.1016/j.pcl.2009.05.016

Vygotsky LS (1962) *Thought and language*. Ed. and trans. Hanfmann E and Vakar G. Cambridge MA: MIT Press.

Wilkinson RG and Pickett K (2009) *The spirit level: Why more equal societies almost always do better*. Bristol: Allen Lane.

Wong ST (2006) The relationship between parent emotion, parent behavior, and health status of young African American and Latino children. *Journal of Pediatric Nursing*, 21(6), 434–42.

World Health Organisation (2009) Women and health: Today's evidence tomorrow's agenda. Geneva: WHO. Retrieved 17 August 2015 from http://whqlibdoc.who.int/publications/2009/9789241563857_eng.pdf

Worldsalaries.org (2008) Professional nurse salaries – international comparison. Retrieved 22 February 2015 from www.worldsalaries.org/professionalnurse.shtml

4 'The *I*, the *Thou* and the *Them*' of children's nursing – Bauman

Introduction

In this chapter I want to explore in greater depth Quine's concept of the *indeterminacy of radical translation* (Murphy 1990: 84) raised in Chapter 2 (p. 26). To recap, Quine states that meaning which is linked to behaviour can only be understood by understanding the group in which it occurs. In Percian pragmatics, we might talk about belief and actions, but essentially the same point is being made. To understand about children's nursing, the meaning of it, or the beliefs which underpin it and which result in the behaviour or action of nurses, we have to understand about the people and the groups who enact children's nursing. Viewed from the outside, as an alien from outer space, the language used in children's nursing would be incomprehensible, the meaning indeterminable. Only by understanding the people who enact children's nursing and how they relate to one another can we understand the meanings they attach to aspects of children's nursing, which affect their actions or behaviours that are part of the phenomena that is children's nursing.

Zagmunt Bauman (1993) has suggested that three modalities exist (Figure 4.1): narcissism where the individual lives for the self; a parasitic state in which the individual lives for the other; and a symbiotic state where the interests of the self and the other are integrated (see also Chapter 5 p. 93).

If we apply these modalities to nursing, the purely narcissistic nurse would be motivated by her or his own needs and desires, such as the need to be appreciated by children and their carers or the desire to be the hero of the day 'saving' the poor little children! The purely parasitic nurse would have no will of their own but

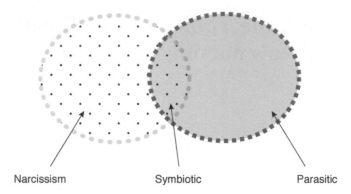

Narcissism   Symbiotic   Parasitic

Figure 4.1 Self and other, after Bauman (1993)

be instead a slave to the requirements of the children and families they look after. It is possible for nurses' narcissism and the parasitic state to merge, where the nurse's desire to be a selfless servant is fulfilled through a slavish devotion to delivering care. However, as Bauman argues, such slavery is immoral, that is, both the slavery which narcissism relies upon, where the narcissist requires others to subjugate their own free will to serve their needs, and the abandonment of free will in the parasitic, which enslaves the person to the will of the other.

A symbiotic state is perhaps then more desirable, where the needs of the nurse and those of children and their carers are all served. However, accepting a symbiotic modality does require that the narcissistic and the parasitic tendencies are acknowledged and held in balance.

Children's nursing is perhaps unique in the family of nursing in that the symbiotic state is played out not just between the nurse and the patient in a sociopolitical culture of healthcare, but in a triad of child–carer (parents)–nurse in a sociopolitical culture of healthcare influenced by a social/cultural understanding of children, childhood and parenting. In children's nursing, the 'I' referred to by Bauman might relate to the nurse, the *thou* would relate to the child and to their carers and the *them* to a form of the other more removed. The *them* here is taken to mean those who organise, resource and evaluate children's nursing – often managers but may also include policy makers and academics.

Set out in this chapter is an attempt to explore the symbiotic relationships which pervade children's nursing in order to understand the dynamics of the groups who generate the meanings attached to children's nursing in the pragmatic belief that such meanings lead to behaviour or actions through which children's nursing is enacted.

The child and the nurse

Many people, nurses included, may like to think that children would thankfully receive nursing care. Romantics may like to imagine that in a postmodern world children nursing is universally welcomed. Unfortunately this is not the case. Children's regard for nurses vary from a positive regard in which the nurse's actions are seen as positive to a negative regard where children always see negative aspects (Randall 2012). The regard children have seems to be unrelated to the actions of the nurse. Thus children's regard might better be described as being towards nurses and nursing, rather than individuals. It appears that children are aware from a very young age that if they require a nurse, they must be ill. Further, that being ill is stigmatised and therefore some degree of what Irving Goffman (1968) termed 'passing' is required (Carnevale 2007).

In passing, people who suffer from a stigmatising condition or illness attempt, either consciously or subconsciously, to conceal or at least not to draw attention to their plight. They attempt to appear to be just like everyone else (without the stigma) in order to interact socially. For adults, passing could be argued to be a social trick or social sleight of hand. However, for children perhaps it performs a more important function as being accepted socially allows children to be part of a childhood cohort which will move through their lifespan together. For children, passing is about maintaining that link to their peers in their community which is vital to living a childhood.

The very presence of a nurse threatens the child's ability to pass – hence why children do not tell their friends when they have a nurse visit them at home, or they have to go to the clinic (Randall 2010). It may also explain why children sometimes find it difficult to talk about nurses and nursing.

In addition, children may not encounter nurses as naive users of healthcare services. Many children who require children's nursing have encountered nurses and other healthcare professionals previously. These encounters may not have been positive, often they will have involved pain, discomfort, loss and perhaps shame and stigma. At each encounter of a nurse and a child, the nurse has to attempt to understand what has gone before in the child's healthcare experience and the effect this 'history' has on the child's attitude towards nurses and nursing. At first this may seem an impossible task: to individually understand each child's experience, to perhaps get each child to recount their past healthcare encounters. However, two factors make the task much easier. One is that children, like adults, generally subscribe to Talcott Parson's (1951) view of the healthcare professional role in the sick role. In Parson's classic sociological explanation, the sick person believes that the nurse participates in the healthcare encounter to help and assist the sick person and not for personal gain or pleasure. Altruism is assumed in order that the sick child, in this case, can trust the nurse and that based on this sense of trust they will divulge information normally considered taboo or socially unacceptable; for example, their bowel habits or sex lives. Children, like adults, understand that nurses are able to access people's bodies in ways other people are not and that allowing such access is not shameful, or socially sanctioned, per se as it would be if one were to allow a stranger or even a lover to access our bodies. Albeit that shame and discomfort may still be associated with the encounter with the nurse, this is often mitigated by reliance on the sick role. Without this level of social compliance, trust and permitted access to bodies it is hard to see how nurses could deliver care, particularly care which supports the practice of medicine (see outcome measure Box 3.1). Acceptance of the sick role in children allows children to face each encounter and tell themselves that while it is not pleasant, it is necessary – a sentiment often reinforced by adults.

The second factor which may help nurses determine the attitude of the child to nursing was referred to in Chapter 3: that nurses through their work build an understanding of the illness process (also of living with disability and life-limiting/threatening conditions). This allows the nurse to build a picture of the events the child is likely to have experienced. Although assumptions can trip us up, we might assume that a child who is coming for a liver transplant assessment has experienced many venopunctures, and other hurtful procedures, and they are likely to be seasoned campaigner, wary but often also resilient.

Through asking children what makes a good nurse (Randall et al. 2008; Randall and Hill 2012) and other studies (Bluebond-Langner 1978), we can see that children have sophisticated understanding of what children's nursing is. While they may not articulate the need to live a childhood as set out in Chapter 3, they do talk about the desire to spend time with their family and friends, that is, to access the environments of childhood (Randall 2011) and the desire that nurses are fun, that is, that they offer play.

Children, like adults, are influenced by the more visible aspects of children's nursing which support the practice of medicine (see Chapter 3, pp. 41–2). When we ask children what do nurses do, not unlike nurses themselves they point most readily to nursing which supports the practice of medicine – the administration of medication (injections), wound care (dressings), monitoring of health status (doing a BP) as a part of monitoring the effectiveness of medical interventions etc. (Randall 2010). Normally the other aspects of children's nursing remain invisible to children, aspects such as facilitating access to education, or a family holiday (Randall 2011), or environments of childhood. As does the border work nurses do ensuring children receive healthcare services such as liaison with other health professionals (Randall 2010). Thus, as William Corsaro (2011) has pointed out, children produce and reproduce the culture in which they live. The peer cultures they produce are in a sense a reproduction of the adult cultures which surround the children. Aspects of the adult culture appear transformed but recognisable in the peer cultures the children enacted. Witness, for example, the sexualised view of nurses demonstrated by young boys:

> A participant wrote on an adhesive note that a 'good nurse' should have: 'Nice buitiful [*sic*] eyes.' And added: 'A nurse to tuck you into bed and give you a kiss.'
>
> (Randall and Hill 2012: 17)

These boys are reproducing the image of nurses portrayed by mass media (Fealy 2004), and often their fathers, for children the sexual image seems less overtly sexual and is often mixed with ideas of the mother and of maternal care.

We should remember, however, that children's regard for nurses (Randall 2012) may not be dependent on the actions of the nurse, or by extension the child's experiences of receiving children's nursing. Rather whether children have a positive or negative regard for nurses may be dependent on the child's own understanding of their illness (Randall 2012). Also we need to be mindful that children living with illness who may require nursing care may have different levels of cognition as a result of the disease or the condition they have. Children may not be particularly conscious of the nurse or of nursing. The concerns set out above about how children regard nurses may be more relevant to situations where children are able to function cognitively, where their internal environment or health status (see Chapter 3) has been stabilised at least to a reasonable extent. In critical or acute care the priority to restore and stabilise the child's health status may become very visible, obscuring the other aspects of children's nursing. The focus on children's nursing supporting the practice of medicine makes the other aspects of children's nursing which facilitate the child's childhood less visible. As pointed out, these aspects might be less visible, but they remain present and important. As the child's cognitive state changes, the issues about how children regard nurses and nursing will move to the foreground (become more important in care landscape, or seem so to children, their carers and/or healthcare workers). For the critically ill child, or any child with altered cognitive state, the focus of care may shift, but the children's nurse need to remain mindful of how children regard nurses and nursing.

The meaning of children's nursing for children is complex, sophisticated and conflicted. Often children have hurtful experiences associated with nurses and nursing, they often recognise that contact with a nurse carries the risk of stigma associated with illness, disability and or life-limiting/threatening conditions. However, children often also recognise that the nurse is acting as a health worker in the social convention of the sick role; indeed, that they as a person living with an illness may rely on the assistance of a nurse to survive.

The nurse and the child

Nurses too may come to children's nursing with a complex set of emotions, motivations and experiences. Nurses are often heard to remark 'I could get the same money with a lot less hassle if I work in...'. What these nurses are saying is that nursing is a job like any other, this might be particular to the UK where managerialism through the 1980s and 1990s has attempted to manage nurses using industrial private sector techniques (Arbuckle 2013). However, in spite of the near constant complaints, these nurses do not leave but continue to nurse. There is then something which despite the stress, the lack of resources and the long hours that keeps nurses in the job.

Nursing as an occupation has been relatively well studied (Witz 1992; Liashencko and Peter 2004) and my intention here is not to discuss why nurses work as nurses, nor the labour politics of nursing, but rather to focus on the meaning children's nurses bring to their work with children and with their carers.

Let us start by trying to define who the '*thou*' is in children's nursing. As we discussed in Chapter 1, adult-focused nursing theories try to define the person in their theorising. While in adult nursing this may be straightforward, in children's nursing the person or the *thou* can be the child as an individual, the child as a member of a family, the carers (parents) of the child, or the family unit as a whole. I have argued in this book that the *thou* we should be talking about is the child as an individual. Taking a stance to relate to the child as an individual is the only stance which can ensure children's rights are taken into account. Taking an individual child stance in the framework of facilitating a childhood allows for the child as a family member to be recognised. It allows nurses to facilitate parenting and to refer to carers for support and help to facilitate their capacity to parent. It also recognises families as a unit in so far as they are integral to a child's childhood and they support the child to live with illness.

However, focusing on the child as an individual living a childhood does not remove all the challenges of defining the relationship of the nurse to the child. Children's nursing demands of nurses a simultaneous juggling of two positions.

The first position is the immersion in the childhoods of the day. To empathise with children and understand their childhoods, children's nurses have to have a working detailed understanding of the current childhood experiences. Ask any children's nurse what the latest trend is in children's culture and they will be able to reel off a list of films, books, TV shows etc. In this sense the *thou* that children's nurses are seeking to serve is the child as a child living a childhood in a particular time and space. To empathise, to understand how the child experiences illness in their communities, the nurse has to in a sense become the *thou*. The *I* becomes the *thou*. Or in less esoteric terms, nurses have to put themselves in the place of the child.

In the second position the nurse acts *in loco parentis* and as a health advisor. They need to see the childhood as it is being lived, but also the childhood as a process which will end and where the child will have to move into adulthood. The immediate gratification of childhood culture may run counter to the child's interests in the longer term and or to their well-being, or health. An example might be that playing video games all night may earn a child kudos with his peers, which might be very important for those isolated by illness, but it is also setting up poor sleep hygiene and the excessive tiredness may compromise the child's immune response and expose them to other increased health risks (Blask 2009).

A further complication is that the 'I' referred to here suggests an individual. However, children's nursing is not a lone sport, but a team game. The *I* then should perhaps more properly be considered as an *'us'* in children's nursing. If we are taking a pragmatic approach, we need to recognise the plurality of children's nurses in time and space (see Chapter 2). Pragmatism does not assume one reality but that many realities coexist. In a pragmatic view there is not a rarefied hegemonic view of children's nursing, or one accepted view, but a pluralistic negotiation of many views, with points of difference, and also points of agreement. For clarity we will stick to *I*, *thou* and *them*, but we should remember that the *I* is one individual's view in a team who deliver care, where the individual nurses may hold different and potentially conflicting views. For example, on the spiritual nature of children's nursing, one nurse may hold religious views and others may be atheists.

If as outlined above, there is a sense in which in the symbiotic relationship the nurse or the *I* becomes the *thou* (the child), in that the nurse has to be able to empathise or put themselves in the child's position, albeit with the caveat of being *in loco parentis.* There is also a sense in which the nurse has to become the *them.*

To understand the systems in which care is delivered, nurses have to understand the *them.* Care is delivered in 'human systems', ones which are socially constructed, inherently political and have their own cultures (Arbuckle 2013). The *them,* often cited as the management, pen pushers or bean counters (as derogatory terms), are portrayed as remote, unconnected or other (i.e. *them* not *I* (us) or *thou*). The *them* in healthcare are often conjured into a spectre to unite teams. In children's nursing, the mantra is often of 'our fight' against the management/system to get children what they need (see Carter 2009, although this is about research, similar arguments are made). Such a narrative is powerful in bringing children's nurses together. It is of course an unarguable argument. Who is going to declare they want to deny children health or well-being? It is of course a fiction too, most if not all managers and bureaucrats also want to provide children with what they need for health and well-being.

At the same time as maintaining a mythology of *us* (nurses) against *them* (managers etc.), nurses also understand that their own advancement in the system, even their continued employment, is dependent on the very people they classify as *them.* To receive promotion or to secure their own position/salary, nurses have to understand the *them.*

On a less mercenary note, the nurse may also be aware that to secure what children need requires an understanding of the people and systems that allocate resources and sustain systems and resources in order to secure the best deal from the system for the children in their care. The nursing team and the *them* of management will always be in a degree of conflict. The managers etc. need to allocate resources and organise systems to deliver care to all children who access a service, or who could potentially access a service. While the individual 'I' nurse is concerned with individual children who may or may not be the priority for those allocating and organising resources and systems. Neither party can deliver care without the other. Managers need individual nurses to deliver care, they could never hope to deliver all the care themselves and individual nurses need the resources and the organisation that managers facilitate to deliver care to individual children.

Within the symbiotic state set out in the introduction to this chapter (p. 66), when the nurse attempts to take on the stance of either the *thou* or the *them*, there are inherent risks. If the nurse over-identifies with the child, they risk becoming, as Bauman states, a slave to the child's needs and losing the free will of their own. If the nurse aligns themself too much with the *them*, they may have a meteoric rise through the organisation, but they risk losing sight of the individual children and of the foundation myths or mission of children's nursing (Arbuckle 2013). I would argue they also risk losing sight of individual children's childhoods and may fail to act to facilitate children's childhoods such that the child living with illness, disability or a life-limiting condition may lose their childhoods.

Gerald Arbuckle (2013: 48) has described a weak group/weak grid culture which may help nurses to negotiate the complexities of the symbiotic state in organisations delivering care to children. In the weak group/weak grid culture, the focus of the team is on the task at hand. In this case the team would focus on improving the lives of children by facilitating their access to their childhood. The status of individuals and the rules or grid structures of the team are less important: they remain in place to give the team cohesion, but they do not prevent creativity, they do not get in the way of finding innovative solutions to complex problems often presented by children who are ill and trying to live a childhood. Such a culture also allows nurses to work with others outside the healthcare team – the group ethos is not so strong as to prevent such cross-agency, cross-discipline working. This sort of multi- and interdisciplinary working is key to facilitating children's childhoods which are lived in communities not in hospitals.

Nurse–child–carer triad

It may be helpful here to revisit Figure 2.2 in Chapter 2 which set out the following possible combinations of the interactions or scenarios between nurse, child and carers:

A Child understanding does not match carers or nurses, e.g. peer cultures

B Carers' understanding does not match child's or nurses, e.g. adult agendas
C The child and nurse share understanding, but carers do not, e.g. supported self-management
D The carer and nurse share understanding, but the child does not, e.g. therapeutic holding
E Carer and child share understanding, but the nurse does not, e.g. family history
F Child, carer and nurse share understanding (desired state)
G Nurse understanding not shared with child nor carers (much of nursing literature and professional agendas).

Points A and B are perhaps more appropriately dealt with under the section below on communities. Point C relates more to the nurse–child interaction described above, as it does not include the carer in any substantial role. Points D–F can be seen as types of interaction between the nurse–child–carer. Point G relates more to the nurse in organisations, and as such is dealt with in the next section.

Scenario D where the nurse and the child's carer share understanding perhaps reflects the often adocentric aspects of societies. Healthcare is designed, funded, enacted and evaluated not by children but by adults. Adult members of societies decide what healthcare children receive (by and large). Despite some challenges to the passive role of children who receive healthcare (Coyne 2008; Moules 2009) and the more general movement to involve users of healthcare including on some occasions children (Salinas 2007), the balance of power in healthcare, as in many aspects of life, remains with adults. It is adult tax dollars/pounds that pay for children's healthcare. It is adult managers/commissioners and bureaucrats who make decisions; albeit they may consult children, they can easily ignore the views of children.

Even at a more day-to-day level, children are disadvantaged by the ways in which adults think about children and childhood. The pre-sociological views of children set out by James et al. (1998: 3–22) can still be found in commonly expressed views about children and in media portrayals. These various views of children suggest that they are incompetent adults and that they lack cognitive and physical skills to function in the adult world, as adults, despite a great deal of work which suggests that children are active participants in their social worlds and that these social worlds interact with the adult cultures in which they are located (Corsaro 2011; Mayal 2008; Prout 2001). This view of children as incompetent may lead to nurses and carers ignoring the child's views and sometimes their human rights (Kelly et al. 2012). The recent work of sociologists and educationalist (Corsaro 2011; Clarke 2005) suggests an emancipatory approach in which children are placed in charge of their own education or, in our case, healthcare.

There are, however, some challenges to such an emancipatory approach in healthcare. While children in schools and preschools are generally well and enjoy reasonable good health, the children we are considering here are living with illness, disability and/or life-limiting/threatening conditions. Children in schools have reasonably stable health status which allows on the whole for reasonably stable cognitive development and acquisition of skills. Children who are living with illness have by definition fluctuating health states which may lead to changes in their cognitive states and affect their abilities to acquire skills (Taylor et al. 2008; see discussion in Chapter 3). For people living with illness there are conditions under which they are unable to make decisions for themselves, such as when unconscious, and this applies to children as it does to adults. The challenge for nurses and children's carers is how to maximise the abilities of children to participate in their healthcare, and how to make judgements as to when and how a proxy view is to be sought (see Chapter 5, 'Ethical symmetries'). To do this would require the development and validation of tools which assess the child's ability to make decisions, including assessing cognitive states in illness, and understanding of illness and of consequences of proposed interventions (as far as they can be determined). Such a tool may also include an assessment of the carer's abilities to act as a proxy decision maker. As yet this children's health decision-making tool does not exist and its development would be an interesting process of negotiating child psychology, paediatric medicine and parenting politics.

There is a danger in scenario D that the nurse and the child's carer (parents) will collude to *do* nursing to children, which may violate their human rights. Certainly excluding children from their care is not helpful in facilitating self-care. As many more children are living with long-term health conditions and many more are living with such conditions into adulthood (Glendinning et al. 2001; Dobbin and Bye 2003), encouraging self-care even in very young children is becoming a priority in order to establish self-management behaviours for life (Kyngas et al. 1998; Wales et al. 2011). Involving children in decision making when they are living with illness is not easy and an uncritical emancipatory approach may not be appropriate. However, nurses need to be critical of the ways in which children and especially children living with illness are perceived and how these perceptions affect their abilities to be full participants in their own healthcare.

At first it may seem that scenario E, where the child and carer share understanding which the nurse is not party to, may have little to do with nursing. Children and their carers (parents etc.) will have a great deal of prior experiences which bind them together but which a nurse has not shared. These experiences will include ways of coping and living with the illness, disability or life-limiting/threatening condition. Nurses may have their textbooks, journals and procedure manuals, but every child and carer living with an illness will develop their own skills, techniques and understanding. For example, a child with Epidermolysis Bullosa (Varki et al. 2006) will require daily dressings. Carers are taught by nurses how to do this, but just as each nurse does dressings slightly differently, so too the carer will develop their own way. This might be in response to the child, perhaps a certain angle of dressing cuts into their skin when they play football, so the carer is careful to place the bandage in such a way to avoid 'football friction'. Such adjustments to care are both desirable and common. Of course one might also imagine the carer of our child with Epidermolysis Bullosa, distracted in a busy household, struggling to get the children to school and themselves to work, deciding that hand washing was too much effort and justifying it to themselves that the bacteria of the household are all the same. Such a breach of the principles of infection control could of course be fatal to such a child (Varki et al. 2006).

Thus nurses must accept that if they delegate nursing tasks to carers, the carer should be at liberty to adapt and change care appropriately. Again a critical approach is required which considers the principles which underpin care and the interests of the child. Nurses must also accept that children and their carers may well find ways of dealing with living with illness which are superior (for them) to the ways suggested by nursing literature, policy and/or practices.

The majority of parent–child relationships are positive but we must be mindful that this is not always the case. Some relationships between parents or other family members and children are abusive and such abuse must be recognised and dealt with according to the laws of the state in which the nurse practises (Jones et al. 2012; Royal College of Paediatrics and Child Health-RCPCH 2010). As well as the more extreme cases of abusive relationships, children and parents/carers may struggle to maintain their relationship where illness places an added pressure to perhaps more 'normal' challenges of intergenerational relationships (Tillery et al. 2014). There may be an argument that nurses should intervene to support children and young people living with illness in their attempts to repair, build and/or maintain their relationships with their parents, in particular in negotiating the child or young person's participation in their care and other aspects of coping with illness. As discussed in Chapter 3, children's nurses see many cases of children living with illness and can therefore build skills over time to help children to negotiate their participation in care and to help children living with illness to foster positive relationships with their parents or other carers. It would be in line with the pragmatic approach set out in Chapters 2 and 3 for nurses to work with children and with their carers (parents) to help children to maintain and sustain their relationships with their family members as this is an important part of childhood, being, as it is, relational (Mayall 2002). Thus nurses may well have a role to play in scenario E, albeit one in which they influence the participants (children and their carers) directly or indirectly, separately or together while perhaps not directly delivering care.

Scenario F would describe an ideal state in which the triad of nurse–child–carer is balanced and understanding is shared. An ideal state might suggest that the triad relationship forms an essence of children's nursing, a universal reality awaiting discovery and description. However, as Richard Rorty (1996) has discussed, such concepts rely on the philosophy of Plato and Cartesian divide of reality and human representation of reality, which pragmatists appose. In the pragmatic approach such a relationship would be seen as a negotiation, continually in flux and influenced by the social, cultural, political time and space in which it occurs. We should remember that this triad arrangement occurs in the context of teams of nurses, and in healthcare interdisciplinary teams in large organisations often of hospitals and other healthcare institutions (e.g. hospices or community teams). It is somewhat naive and simplistic perhaps to limit the relationships in children's nursing to a triad of nurse–child–carer.

The interactions of nurses, children and their carers may contain aspects of all the scenarios of A–G set out above, or may feature some aspects more than others. This would be in line with the pragmatic approach which considers multiple realities and perspectives in a time and space context (Rorty 1996). This approach may be particularly helpful in considering the nursing of children where the roles of each of the parties will change with the child's health status and over time. Currently the role the nurse should play and when that role should change to facilitate self-care or care by the child's carer is determined more by traditional practices, intuition and experience than by any assessment of the child's capacity or that of their carers to be active participants. A pragmatic approach may be useful in that the judgements made in the nurse–child–carer triad are often subject to prevailing views of children's competence and capacities which may disadvantage children in general, even deny them their human rights, and in particular may disadvantage children living with illness.

The pragmatic approach may be useful in attempting to understand how the relationships between individual nurses (in teams), children and their carers are enacted in healthcare organisations.

The organisation and the nurse

If the interactions of the nurse, the child and their carer are those of the *I* and the *thou*, then by moving to the organisation level we are moving towards the *them*. In considering the organisation of nursing, I am thinking not just of clinical healthcare facilities such as hospitals, hospices, respite facilities and community services, but also of professional/trade union groups, academic educational institutions and regulatory bodies. We might usefully divide these into employment-related organisations and professional-related organisations. Obviously some organisations perform both functions, but often within the organisation there is also a division in similar terms.

First we should remember that although a great deal of healthcare for children is delivered and received informally, what we are concerned with here is the practice of children's nursing, as work done by paid employees. Apart from the rare circumstance of the self-employed children's nurse, in the main nurses work in organisations. The responsibility for delivery of care is often assumed in part at least not by the nurse but by the hospital, hospice or community healthcare provider, through vicarious liability.

Both the status of the nurse as employee and that of the nurse as professional are contested. The contractual arrangements of employee and employer have in general been formed by the practice of capitalism (Arbuckle 2013). They are constructed around the delivery, in this case perhaps, of a service industry. Nurses are employed for a certain number of hours, with overtime payments for exceeding the contractual hours. If one is advising on broadband connection, this works well: the consultation service is advertised as being available for certain hours. The arrangement works less well if one is consoling a child who has realised that their friend from the ward has died from the same condition they have. Admittedly this does not occur every day (thankfully), but as outlined above (Chapter 3, p. 48), the work of nurses is subject to pressures which make containing it within set hours problematic. In addition there are the moral and conceptual challenges characterising the work of nurses with children as equivalent to service industries designed to deliver profits for shareholders. The moral argument we can save for Chapter 5. Conceptually the challenges come in aligning the business of children's nursing with the mission or, as Arbuckle (2013) describes, it the foundation myth. What I am suggesting in this book is that the business of children's nursing has to support and contribute to the facilitation of children's childhoods within their communities. It may be unrealistic to expect children's nurses to overthrow capitalism! But what can be achieved is a realignment of systems and resources to support nurses in their work of facilitating childhoods.

Currently all too often the efforts of nurses to facilitate children living a childhood is fragmented and frustrated by the systems in which they have to work. Particularly for nurses, working in organisations whose primary goal (or foundation myth) may not be the provision of children's healthcare, but rather adult healthcare. Many children's nurses work in organisations which provide adult healthcare and in which children's health provision is a very small part of the organisation's work. In such organisations children's nurses are at a structural disadvantage, the services they deliver represent a very small proportion of the total budget (children's nurses in 2008 made up just 4.23 per cent of registered nurses (Nursing and Midwifery Council 2008), when population estimates indicated child population 0–19 was 24 per cent of the UK population in 2008 (ONS)), and the workforce is small in comparison to adult services. Children's nurses rarely have the critical mass within the organisation to be promoted to senior positions in sufficient numbers to make useful strategic alliances with other children's nurses, or even other children's workers.

As discussed in Chapter 3 (p. 58), facilitating children's childhoods is not just the preserve of nursing or of health. Yet working across disciplinary boundaries and organisations is rarely encouraged or rewarded. More often care is fragmented by cultural professional silos in which groups act to promote and preserve the interests of their professional group (Arbuckle 2013). The group may use a narrative of fighting for children's needs, promoting their professional group's interest in the belief that this is the best way to secure what children need. Where professional groups are working in organisations in competition with other groups, the dynamics of the organisation may leave them little choice but to attempt to secure their own position in order to access resources (see Randall and McKeown 2014).

Children's nurses need to construct and reconstruct children's healthcare such that they work in organisations which have the facilitation of childhoods as its foundation myth or mission statement/vision. The structures and use of resources in such an organisation would support children's nurses to work with colleagues in education and social care, and would extend far beyond the hospital walls.

Our proposed new employer might have the following mission statement:

> We will ensure all children, irrespective of illness, disability or a life-limiting/threatening condition, have a childhood which is equal to that of their peers, in their communities.

The organisation of children's nursing is not limited to employment. Above we outlined scenario G where the understanding of nurses was not shared by the child, or the child's carers. Such concepts might be seen as professional constructs (see Shields et al. 2007, 2012 on family centre care as a professional construct; Coleman 2010). These concepts are created and maintained in education institutions and in the nursing literature, and they are also often endorsed and used by employer organisations such as hospitals (see Birmingham Children's Hospital www.bch.nhs.uk/story/mission-vision-and-values). All these practices are bound together by a concept of a nursing profession. In order for an occupation to frame itself as a profession, the people who undertake it have to establish three things: a body of knowledge, social closure and a social contract (Abbot and Meerabeau 1998). The moral arguments as to whether attempts at social closure are compatible with the social contract of children's nursing will be addressed in Chapter 5. Here I want to focus on the construction of a body of knowledge from a pragmatic perspective.

Despite the romantic idea of the lone thinker/writer generating ideas, it is organisations and institutions which generate and sustain ideas (de Botton 2012). Even in the modern information age, a tweet that goes viral can still not compete with a peer-reviewed paper published in a respected journal. Chiefly because the random internet posting relies on word of mouth, or mouse clicks and is not consistently catalogued, while a peer-reviewed paper is available through thousands of educational institutions, is catalogued in databases such as Pubmed or Proquest, and can be searched for, found and retrieved for decades by anyone with a computer and a little understanding of literature searching (or who knows a friendly librarian).

With the power of information in a digital age and the organisations and institutions which propagate, publish and promote the information come some challenges and restrictions. The problems of peer-review mechanism are well known (Stern and Simes 1997) and not limited to children's nursing, as are the difficulties with reliance on a for-profit share ownership publishing industry (van Noorden 2013). However, for children's nursing the organisation of a body of knowledge presents particular challenges.

At the root of these challenges are the difficulties with critical mass. Globally the proportion of children aged 0–14 as a percentage of the total population varies from 50 per cent to 13 per cent with an average of 28.36 per cent (World Bank 2015). Thus in most populations the number of children's nurses required will be less than for the adult population even if the proportion of children's nurses matched the child population. The number of children's nurses is likely to be small in proportion to other nurses (see above in 2008 only 4.23 per cent of registered nurses were children's nurses in the UK (NMC 2008)). The number available to undertake further education and to develop writing skills and research skills is also likely to be small. In addition, the number of people interested in reading about children's nursing is equally likely to be small. Unfortunately academic outcome measures internationally are based very largely on crude measures of number. Academics are measured by their publications in terms of impact. A journal attracts a higher impact factor based on the number of citations of the papers it carries: an academic's H factor, a measure of their influence, is based on how many times they are cited by others (Jackson et al. 2009). With a smaller pool to draw on, children's nursing academics cannot generate H factors to equal their adult colleagues. Journals dedicated to children's healthcare have much lower impact factors than journals which may carry some child-related papers, but which are aimed at a much wider readership. As Figure 4.2 shows, the impact factor for paediatric journals (aggregated five-year impact factor of 3.416 in JCR 2012 Science Edition ISI Web of Knowledge) is much lower than that of general and internal (adult) medicine (aggregated five-year impact factor of 38.835 (Thompson Reuters 2014)).

Like children's nurses employed in organisations where the main concern is providing adult healthcare, academics who want to develop careers in children's nursing face similar problems of competing with more numerous adult-focused colleagues in an environment structurally weighted in favour of adult nursing. There are many more student nurse places for adult-focused nursing, many more units or modules of study focused on adult healthcare to be taught in programmes.

It is hardly surprising that children's nursing lacks a well-developed academic body of understanding. By refocusing children's nursing to facilitate childhoods, nursing academics could make common cause with academics from other disciplines in education and social care. The appeal of their work may reach a larger readership increasing the impact of their work. However, in addition, it seems likely that children's nursing academics will need to organise to challenge current success measures in academia. A start might be to devise and evaluate outcome measures for academics which facilitate inter-disciplinary work and value a contribution to improving children's lives as well as the generation of understanding about children's nursing. These measures need to be championed within universities

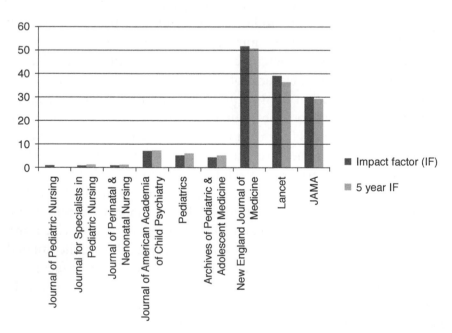

Figure 4.2 Impact factors top three journals for children's nursing, paediatrics vs general and internal medicine

Source: adapted from 2012 JCR Science Edition ISI Web of Knowledge, Thompson Reuters (2014).

to ensure wide-scale acceptance and adoption of the measures, such that academics can move between institutions and have their work valued in similar terms. Shifting the outcome measures in this way will be a long-term and challenging project, but if the complexities of children's nursing are to be addressed and solutions devised, implemented and evaluated, then a cooperative, long-term strategy is required.

Communities

Community is a concept which is often difficult to define, but which like culture is one which is recognisable to people who have experienced it. Communities might be seen as *I*, *thou* or as *them*, the degree of otherness being dependent on the degree of empathy or identification the nurse has with the community in question. The nurse may be a member of or understand well communities seen as *I* or *thou*, while *them* might be applied to people from communities stigmatised or strange.

The way 'communities' are anthropomorphised into single identities, as though they were a single person, of course belies the way in which many views, perspectives and understandings are contained within any community. However, alongside the differences in communities are also commonalities, which can be helpful in understanding the way children's nursing is constructed.

Part of the pragmatic approach set out in Chapter 3 (p. 54) is the consideration of the influence of culture on children's childhoods as lived in a time and space (Chapter 2). When we consider how communities understand children's nursing, we have to consider the potential conflicts as well as the potential synergies between elements within communities, and between communities. In some communities the child's carer may receive substantial support, both material and psychological, from neighbours who consider the carer to be a member of their community. However, if the carer does not attend to the social codes of the community, perhaps because they are attempting to cope with an ill child, then they may be rejected and at best support withdrawn, at worst the child and family may be victimised and driven out of the neighbourhood, with the associated disruption to nursing care.

The parenting of children does not occur just in family groups, but also in neighbourhoods and communities. Parents seek and may receive support, information and material help from others who are parents, or who have experience of parenting (Findler 2008). These sources of support etc. in communities may be geographically located close to the family or may be separated by in some cases considerable distances and time. Grandparents may influence the health practices of the child's carers, but may be living in another part of the country, abroad or even influence from beyond the grave, via practice and beliefs handed down through families.

As we discussed in Chapter 3, if nurses are to facilitate childhoods for children living with illness, part of this is to ensure children experience the relationships in their communities, as childhood is relational (Mayall 2002). Thus children's nurses need to encourage and support community involvement. Part of the assessment of parental capacity suggested in outcome measure 3.5 should include how the child's carers access support from their community and how they connect and allow their children to connect with their community. The caveats set out in outcome measure 3.6 also need to be borne in mind.

Working with community leaders both at the individual level and at the strategic level where ideas and policies are created and resources allocated may help children's nurses to build alliances. As in many other areas of children's healthcare, the number of children's nurses who operate at a strategic level is likely to be small (see argument for academics above). Building alliances with community leaders and colleagues in education and social care is then important in influencing the public health and children's health and well-being agendas. This would apply as much on an international scale as it would on national and more local levels.

The discussion thus far perhaps addresses scenario B from above: we think of children's carers as being members of a community and sharing that community's understanding in ways perhaps not fully shared by children or nurses. As discussed in Chapter 3, the individual challenges carers might face (such as drug addiction) and which affect their capacity to care for the child would need to be addressed by children's nurses by referral to appropriate adult services. Many of these problems might be seen as social problems within communities, however, the same arguments as those used at the individual level would apply: that children's nurses raise awareness of the effects on children's health, but that they call on those responsible to take action, rather than attempting to address the social problem themselves.

Finally there is scenario A where the child's understanding is not matched by that of either the nurse or their carer. This might occur in peer cultures or communities. As already identified by William Corsaro (2011), in peer cultures children produce and reproduce a culture. Corsaro gives some charming examples of how the banking crisis of 2008 is used by children in their play. In healthcare, Myra Bluebond-Langner's (1978) account of the trading of white cell counts in the oncology ward serves as a similar example of how children take aspects of adult cultures, in which they live, and use them in their own way.

The phenomena of passing and the importance of experiencing a childhood along with one's peers as discussed in Chapter 2 mean that peer cultures are very influential in affecting children's health behaviours. As Kyngas et al. (1998) have shown with diabetic control, nurses can explore peer cultures with children and adapt their advice to the child's experiences in the peer culture to improve health. Scenario A should not then be allowed to persist; it is the work of children's nurses to seek to understand healthcare from the child's perspectives – to work with children to explore their meanings of children's nursing.

Summary

Because of radical interpretation we need to understand how those who participate in children's nursing understand children's nursing. Standing outside we cannot hope to understand the meaning and therefore the actions taken by those who participate in children's nursing. This is not an easy task, as this group includes children, their carers, the communities they live in, nurses and various stakeholder organisations and institutions, all of whom have different views and different agendas.

However, there are commonalities both within these groups and between these groups. The pragmatic approach allows us to take account of these different views, to place them in a context of a time and space and to explore the conflicts and synergies. Using a critical approach allows nurses to consider the social status of children and of children's nursing to understand how this may affect nurses facilitating a childhood for children living with illness.

For clarity I have separated out the moral and ethical aspects in this discussion and will turn to these in the next chapter. It could be argued that the dynamics of the symbiotic relationship between *I, thou* and *them* discussed above cannot be separated in this way from the political, ethical and moral judgements which are made in delivering or not delivering children's nursing.

References

Abbott P and Meerabeau L (1998) Professionals, professionalization and the caring professions. In Abbott P and Meerabeau L (eds) *The sociology of the caring professions*, 2nd edn (pp. 1–19). London: UCL Press.

Arbuckle GA (2013) *Humanising healthcare reforms*. London: Jessica Kingsley.

Bauman Z (1993) The moral party of two. In Bauman Z (ed.) *Postmodern ethics* (pp. 82–109). Oxford: Blackwell.

Blask DE (2009) Melatonin, sleep disturbance and cancer risk. *Sleep Medicine Reviews*, 13(4), 257–64. doi:10.1016/j.smrv.2008.07.007

Bluebond-Langner M (1978) *The private worlds of dying children*. Princeton: Princeton University Press.

Carnevale FA (2007) Revisiting Goffman's stigma: The social experience of families with children requiring mechanical ventilation at home. *Journal of Child Health Care*, 11(1), 7–18.

Carter B (2009) Tick box for child? The ethical positioning of children as vulnerable, researchers as Barbarians and reviewers as overly cautious. *International Journal of Nursing Studies*, 46(6), 858–64. doi:10.1016/j.ijnurstu.2009.01.003

Clark A (2005) Ways of seeing using the Mosaic approach to listen to young children's perspectives. In Clark A, Trine Kjorholt A and Moss P (eds) *Beyond listening children's perspectives on early child hood services* (pp. 29–51). Bristol: Policy Press.

Coleman V (2010) The evolving concept of family centred care. In Smith L and Coleman V (eds) *Child and family-centred healthcare: Concept, theory and practice*, 2nd edn (pp. 1–26). Basingstoke: Palgrave Macmillan.

Corsaro WA (2011) *The sociology of childhood*, 3rd edn. Thousand Oaks, CA: Pine Forge Press/Sage.

Coyne I (2008) Children's participation in consultations and decision making at health service level: A review of the literature. *International Journal of Nursing Studies*, 45(11), 1682–9. doi: 10.1016/j.ijnurstu.2008.05.002

de Botton A (2012) Institutions. In de Botton A (ed.) *Religion for atheists: A non-beliver's guide to the uses of religion* (pp. 277–315). London: Hamish Hamilton.

Dobbin CJ and Bye PTP (2003) Clinical perspectives: Adults with cystic fibrosis: Meeting the challenge! *Internal Medicine Journal,* 33(12), 593–7.

Glendinning C, Kirk S, Guliffrida A and Lawton D (2001) Technology dependent children in the community definition, numbers and costs. *Child Care Health and Development,* 27(4), 321–34.

Goffman E (1968) *Stigma: Notes on the management of spoiled identity.* Harmondsworth: Penguin.

Fealy GM (2004) 'The good nurse': Visions and values in images of the nurse. *Journal Advanced Nursing,* 46(6), 649–56.

Findler L (2008) Support behind the scenes: Attitudes and practice of pediatricians and nurses with grandparents of sick children. *Family and Community Health,* 31(4), 317–25.

Jackson D, Haigh C and Watson R (2009) Editorial: Nurses and publications – the impact of the impact factor. *Journal of Clinical Nursing,* 18(18), 2537–8 doi: 10.1111/j.1365–2702.2009.02927.x

James A, Jenks C and Prout A (1998) *Theorizing childhood.* Cambridge: Polity Press.

Jones L, Bellis MA, Wood S, Hughes K, McCoy E, Eckley L, Bates G, Mikton C, Shakespeare T and Office A (2012) Prevalence and risk of violence against children with disabilities: A systematic review and meta-analysis of observational studies. *The Lancet,* 380(9845), 899–907. doi: 10.1016/S0140–6736(12)60692–8

Kelly M, Jones S, Wilson V and Lewis P (2012) How children's rights are constructed in family-centred care: A review of the literature. *Journal of Child Health Care,* 16(2), 190–205. doi: 10.1177/1367493511426421

Kyngas H, Hentinen M and Barlow JH (1998) Adolescents' perceptions of physicians, nurses, parents and friends: Help or hindrance in compliance with diabetes self care? *Journal of Advanced Nursing,* 27(4), 760–9.

Liaschenko J and Peter E (2004) Nursing ethics and conceptualisations of nursing: Profession, practice and work. *Journal of Advanced Nursing,* 46(5), 488–95.

Mayall B (2002) *Towards a sociology for childhood: Thinking from children's lives.* Birmingham: Open University Press.

Mayall B (2008) Conversations with children: Working with generational issues. In Christensen P and James A (eds) *Research with children: Perspectives and practices,* 2nd edn (pp. 109–25). Abingdon: Routledge.

Moules T (2009) 'They wouldn't know how it feels': characteristics of quality care from young people's perspectives: A participatory research report. *Journal of Child Health Care,* 13(4), 322–33. doi: 10.1177/1367493509344824

Murphy PJ (1990) *Pragmatism from Peirce to Davidson.* Boulder, CO: West View Press.

van Noorden R (2013) The true cost of science publishing: Cheap open-access journals raise questions about the value publishers add for their money. *Nature,* 495 (28 March), 426–9.

Nursing and Midwifery Council (2008) Statistical analysis of the register 1 April 2007 to 31 March 2008. Retrieved 22 February 2015 from www.nmc-uk.org/Documents/Statistical%20analysis%20of%20the%20register/NMC-Statistical-analysis-of-the-register-2007–2008.pdf

Office of National Statistics (2008) National population projections 2008-based. Series PP2 No 27, ONS. Retrieved 17 August 2015 from http://www.ons.gov.

uk/ons/rel/npp/national-population-projections/2008-based-projections/national-population-projections.pdf

Parsons T (1951) *The social system.* London: Routledge and Kegan Paul.

Prout A (2001) Representing children: Reflections on the children 5–16 programme. *Children and Society,* 15(3), 193–201. doi: 10.1002/chi.667

Randall D (2010) 'They just do my dressings': Children's perspectives on community children's nursing. Unpublished PhD thesis, University of Warwick, Warwick.

Randall D (2011) 'To be like the others': Children's views of nursing in community settings. In Brykczynska G and Simons J (eds) *Ethical and philosophical aspects of nursing children and young people* (pp. 77–87). Oxford: Blackwell.

Randall D (2012) Children's regard for nurses and nursing: A mosaic of children's views on community nursing. *Journal of Child Health Care,* 16(1), 91–104. doi: 10.1177/1367493511426279

Randall D and Hill A (2012) Consulting children and young people on what makes a good nurse. *Nursing Children and Young People,* 24(3), 14–19.

Randall D and McKeown M (2014) Editorial: Failure to care: Nursing in a state of liquid modernity? *Journal of Clinical Nursing,* 23(5–6), 766–7. doi: 10.1111/jocn.12441

Randall D, Stammers P and Brook G (2008) Asking children how to make good children's nurses. *Paediatric Nursing,* 20(5), 22–6.

Rorty R (1996) Introduction: Relativism: Finding and making. In Rorty R (ed.) *Philosophy and social hope* (pp. xvi–xxxii). London: Penguin.

Royal College of Paediatrics and Child Health-RCPCH (2010) *Safeguarding children and young people: Roles and competences for health care staff. Intercollegiate document.* London: Royal College of Paediatrics and Child Health.

Salinas E (2007) *Evaluation study of the staying positive pilot workshops: A self management programme for young people with chronic conditions.* Oxford: Expert Patient Programme, University of Oxford.

Shields L, Pratt J, Davis L and Hunter J (2007) Family-centred care for children in hospital. *Cochrane Database Systematic Reviews* 2007 (CD004811). doi: 10.1002/14651858.CD004811.pub2

Shields L, Zhou H, Pratt J, Taylor M, Hunter J and Pascoe E (2012) Family-centred care for hospitalised children aged 0–12 years. *Cochrane Database of Systematic Reviews,* 10 (CD004811). doi: 10.1002/14651858.CD004811.pub3

Stern JM and Simes RJ (1997) Publication bias: Evidence of delayed publication in a cohort study of clinical research projects. *British Medical Journal,* 315(13), 640–5.

Taylor RM, Gibson F and Franck LS (2008) The experience of living with a chronic illness during adolescence: A critical review of the literature. *Journal of Clinical Nursing,* 17(23), 3083–91 doi: 10.1111/j.1365–2702.2008.02629.x

Tillery R, Long A and Phipps S (2014) Child perceptions of parental care and overprotection in children with cancer and healthy children. *Journal of Clinical Psychology in Medical Settings,* 21(2), 165–72. doi: 10.1007/s10880–014–9392–5

Thompson Reuters (2014) 2012 JCR Science Edition ISI Web of Knowledge. Retrieved 22 February 2015 from http://about.jcr.incites.thomsonreuters.com/

Varki R, Sadowski S, Pfender E and Uitto J (2006) Epidermolysis Bullosa.1. Molecular genetics of the junctional and hemidesmosomal variants. *Journal of Medical Genetics,* 43(8), 641–52.

Wales S, Crisp J, Fernandes R and Kyngas H (2011) Modification and testing of the chronic disease compliance instrument to measure treatment compliance in adolescents with asthma. *Contemporary Nurse*, 39(2), 147–56.

Witz A (1992) *Professions and patriarchy*. London: Routledge.

World Bank (2015) Data: Population ages 0–14 (% of total). Retrieved 22 February 2015 from http://data.worldbank.org/indicator/SP.POP.0014.TO.ZS

5 What's the good of children's nursing?

Introduction

> The true is the name of whatever proves itself to be good in the way of belief, and good too for definite, assignable reason.
>
> (James quoted by Murphy 1990: 56)

A central plank of pragmatism is what works is good, and what is good works. A common retort to this is: 'Works for whom?' 'And in what sense works?' (Rorty 1996a). These are the themes of this chapter. First using a framework of ethical symmetries to explore whether children's nursing should operate to different ethics and moral standards than those used in the nursing care of adults, then using Urban Walker's expressive collaborative morality to discuss the allocation of responsibilities for children's nursing.

Before we begin we should address a prominent criticism of pragmatism and pragmatists, which is that they rely on relativism (Rorty 1996b). All the views of children's nursing discussed in Chapters 3 and 4 are held as equally valid and not valid. Using a pragmatic approach one cannot claim to have the 'right' approach (even the pragmatic approach taken here to facilitating childhoods is not claimed as being definitive). Pragmatism rejects the Cartesian divide, the dualism of something being right (i.e. that it exists outwith social constructions and has a truth which is constant) and other things being wrong (i.e. they are perceptions of a reality which have been misinterpreted or misconstructed by people). Rather, as Richard Rorty (1996b) explains, the best we might achieve is to understand how ideas work in a time and space for particular groups of people.

Rorty (1996a) adds that this pragmatic understanding may or may not serve the moral and ethical or political ideals of a society. Or as Rorty puts it, justice and reality may coincide but they may not, there is no unified universal just reality. There is no ideal way of doing children's nursing which will fit all times and all children, in all communities. For our purposes here we might want to consider that there are ways in which children's nursing is practice, and then there are aspirations of children, their carers and nurses as to how they would like children's nursing to be. It is possible that the practice of children's nursing matches the aspirations, but it is also possible it does not, that it is constructed by other groups, such as bureaucrats under pressure to cut costs. For Rorty (1996a) ideas are tools. One can use the concepts of children's nursing to help children live a childhood or to shut a local hospital. The ideas are not to blame; the people using them in a particular time and space are responsible for their actions and the results. Rorty (1996a) uses this concept of ideas to justify drawing on the work of Martin Heidegger, claiming his ideas are useful despite his membership of the Nazi party and Heidegger declaring himself the Fuhrer of Heidelberg University (Sheehan 1988). Rorty was also heavily influenced by John Dewey, a lifelong social democrat.

The pragmatic approach allows us to examine ideas about children's nursing in a historical context. Rather than debating whether restricting parental visiting was right or wrong, pragmatists look at how the ideas were used in a time and space (or cultural context), who did these ideas work for and how. Looked at through a pragmatist lens we might discuss how restricted parental visiting was used by the developing children's nursing profession to lay claim to the work of caring for children living with illness, a role previously reserved for mothers in the home. That such ideas would be abhorrent now to parents, children and many nurses is not the point. At that time, in that space, they worked to professionalise children's nursing.

To be clear, pragmatism does not make ethical and moral decisions for us, it merely allows us to examine who children's nursing works for and in what ways in a particular time and space. This is not to suggest that the ethical and moral decisions are not important, which they are, but that they are political and cultural matters rather than ones of universal principle. What I outline below are two approaches to these political and cultural matters which may be helpful to children's nurses.

Ethical symmetries

In many societies childhood and children are held as 'special'. Although there may be some good reasons for this cultural value being attached to childhood, it can also alienate and isolate children from other members of the society. Being cast as a special case can be something of a double-edged sword. The approach of ethical symmetries as outlined by Christenson and Prout (2002) offers a way to connect children with the adult majority in a society.

As Randall et al. (2013) have pointed out, there are a number of asymmetries in societies which affect the health of children. Asymmetries or inequalities by definition privilege one group in a society over another. Christensen and Prout (2002) have used the work of Zagmunt Bauman (1993) (discussed in Chapter 4) to set out their argument that those in the majority group might be considered the *I* and those in minority groups considered the other (*thou* or *them*). Christensen and Prout (2002) suggest that a distinction can be made, based on Bauman's analysis between taking responsibility *away* from children and taking responsibility *for* children. They infer that taking responsibility *away* from children is akin to a paternalistic approach where adults make decisions instead of children. This would perhaps match scenario D discussed in Chapters 2 and 4 where children's nursing is done to children rather than *with* them, where nurses and carers do not share their understanding with the child in ways they can understand, but often with force impose nursing on children (RCN 2010). Christensen and Prout agree with Bauman that the minority (*thou* or *them*) should not be treated the same as the majority group, nor should the minority group (in our case children) be considered a homogenous entity. This means that statements like 'They are only six they won't understand' should not be used, as it assumes that all six years olds have a common level of understanding. When in fact six year olds differ in their levels of understanding, in particular there is some evidence that young children who have experienced illness develop skills and understanding which are not seen in those not exposed to illness (Khair et al. 2013)

Rather, Christensen and Prout declare in taking responsibility *for* children involves

> entering a dialogue that recognises commonality but also honours difference.
>
> (2002: 408)

A point echoed in many aspects of this book (see Chapter 2) and in pragmatics more generally (Rorty 1996b). Seeking ethical symmetry is about treating children living with illness as equal members of societies, not about treating them the same as everyone else. As Randall et al. (2013) point out, ethical symmetry is not ethical parity.

Christensen and Prout (2002) have suggested two processes which might aid nurses to achieve ethical symmetry. The first process is to examine their own assumptions about children and childhood. Many of these assumptions are examined in Chapter 2 where we considered the temporal and relational aspects of childhoods. Here a word of warning may be appropriate: many of our assumptions about children are based on developmental models (Blackford 2004). In line with the pragmatic approach, these understandings, which were once held as 'true', should be critically examined and we should be prepared to find them fallible. There is now a great deal of debate on many aspects of these developmental models (James et al. 1998). As Randall et al. (2013) have suggested, it may be more helpful to discover the abilities of each child in the context rather than to rely on developmental models. They also suggest the use of reflexive questions which might aid the nurse in examining their assumptions such as:

> Would I treat an adult in this way? ... Would I treat a well, rich child from a majority community in this way?
>
> (2013: 18, 19)

As Randall et al. (2013) point out, answering 'no' is as valid as answering 'yes'. The point is to justify the ethical symmetry, to examine one's assumptions. There may well be good reasons for treating children and adults differently (Christensen and Prout 2002). To achieve ethical symmetry between rich and poor children, these groups may well need to be treated differently (Randall et al. 2010).

The second process suggested by Christensen and Prout (2002) is to place the justification of children's ethical symmetry in a political/ cultural context. Or as pragmatists might say, in time and space. In adult care we might expect the person to be responsible for aspects of their care such as keeping outpatients appointments and knowing what medication they are taking. In taking responsibility *for* children, we might be concerned if no adults in their life were supporting the child to manage aspects of their healthcare. It might not be possible for children to use transport to attend outpatients appointments. Often children do not have access to an income, so may just not be able, like adults, to afford the fare. As set out in Chapter 3, facilitating self-care in children is a part of children's nursing, but so is protecting children from neglect and abuse. As is perhaps indicated in this example, we need to consider the position of children in families and communities both on an individual level and on a social or population level.

Taking responsibility *for* children using ethical symmetry is a political stance. It assumes that children are a minority disadvantaged group. In 2009–13 the proportion of the total population aged 0–14 for countries covered by the World Bank/UN data (2015) ranged from 50 per cent Niger–49 per cent Chad to 12 per cent Hong Kong and Macao (China)–13 per cent Germany, Japan and Qatar (with a global average of 28.36 per cent). Generally children make up a sizable minority (just) in majority or developing countries with low to average incomes, while they are a much smaller minority in numbers terms in higher income countries. Some have also challenged the view of children as passive disadvantaged members of societies (James et al. 1998; Mayall 2002), pointing to how children are active members, producing and reproducing their own cultures which influence majority adult culture as much as they in turn are influenced by adult culture (Corsaro 2011).

We should remember, however, that here we are considering children living with illness, disability and life-limiting/threatening conditions. The view of these children as passive is also contended (Admi 1995) but the case of these children as a minority disadvantage group is stronger because illness, disability and life-limiting/threatening conditions isolate children and disadvantage them and their families in several ways (Department of Education and Skills and HM Treasury 2007); for example, by limiting parental incomes and or work advancement because of the demands of caring for a child placed on parents who also work. Social and structural disadvantage or asymmetries arise for a child and their family from a child's illness. Arguably not because of the child's illness per se, but from social construction of and reaction to the child's illness (Kearney and Pryor 2004). This again perhaps explains why children living with illness wish to 'pass' to appear to be like other children not living with illness (Carnevale 2007; Randall 2011). It also raises an ethical dilemma. Do the attempts of nurses to cast children and their carers as disadvantaged, as victims of ethical asymmetries undermine the child and their carers' attempts at passing, at appearing as not disadvantaged by illness or disability? Pragmatics help us to understand that for nurses ethical symmetries might work (in a particular political space and time) to advance a view of nurses as defenders of children and families, avengers of the disadvantaged. However, such strategies can work against the child and their carers' need to pass. For children and their carers, an agenda to achieve equity to have a childhood, as equal to that of their peers in their community, might help to support their passing.

Here we have to grasp the interconnection that the pragmatist rejection of Cartesian dualism entails: the political stance to address ethical symmetries or not to do so, both are a part of children's nursing. As Richard Rorty puts it, 'we insist that human belief cannot swing free of the nonhuman environment' (1996b: 32). So how we talk about children, childhoods, illness and nursing, the language we use are all a part of the phenomena of children's nursing. Taking a political stance or not taking one are both political acts which reflect beliefs about children, about childhood and about in this case illness and nursing. Thinking and talking about children's nursing as addressing ethical symmetries is a political stance and, if adopted, changes children's nursing. However, what it does not do is determine who is responsible for the actions to address ethical symmetries. To address that question we need to turn to the work of Margaret Urban Walker (2007).

Children's nursing a moral endeavour – Margaret Urban Walker

It should be of no surprise by now that I want to claim Margaret Urban Walker as a pragmatist. Her book on moral understanding is a feminist work, but recognises women's voices in a pluralist sense as many voices. Walker proposes that moral understanding only occurs within a social context. Like Davidson and other pragmatists, she sees moral understanding being contained within the human social context in which it occurs, rather than relying on universal principles. In line with the views of other pragmatists, Walker's expressive collaborative morality is anti-Cartesian: it is made by people and between people, it does not exist as a separate reality waiting to be found (Rorty 1996b).Walker's discussion of how moral responsibility is accepted or rejected is action-orientated, concerned with the ethics of social interactions in what people do. She considers the beliefs which lead to ethical actions just as a pragmatist considers the actions which arise from belief (Murphy 1990).

Walker says of her expressive collaborative model:

> Like all interpretive devices, this model is a creature of its specific historical time and social place.
>
> (Walker 2007: 67)

Walker proposes the expressive collaborative model in opposition to a theoretical judicial model. While in her alternative the moral discussion is articulated between people to describe and critique moral understanding, in the theoretical judicial model male elites prescribe moral understanding and enforce these onto others. Walker argues that by imposing the moral understanding of the elites the moral understanding of others in a society are hidden. Her proposed expressive collaborative model uncovers the voices of those in societies who do not hold power, and she argues for a collaborative approach in which the taking and the rejecting of responsibilities is negotiated within social groups. There are obvious parallels between Walker's ideas on expressive collaborative morality and John Dewey's ideas on education as a democratic process. Dewey considers two points key:

How numerous and varied are the interest which are consciously shared? How full and free is the interplay with other forms of association?

(1944: 83)

Dewey argues that in democratic states ideas have to be shared between the executive and the electorate in order that representation and decisions can be made, and policies and practices followed. In terms of healthcare, the democratic tradition would suggest that patients (children), their carers and the multidisciplinary team all have something to offer, rather than a reliance on a single elite group such as the medical profession. Such a view could be argued to have become the consensus in the past few years with recognition of the failings of a patronising and deferential culture which was perhaps typified by 1950s medical hegemony (Freidson 1970) and with the introduction of ideas such as expert patients (Salinas 2007) and patient public involvement (DH 2002). Dewey's and Walker's ideas are not just important because they come from a liberal Western tradition, as does healthcare itself, but because numerous shared ideas are much more likely to offer the solutions to the complex challenges of children's diseases and healthcare than narrow ideas rigidly imposed. Hence the move to open access publishing which allows much wider access to research and scholarship (Finch Group 2013). Dewey also warns that where education is limited, perhaps to a mode more akin to 'training', where the interconnection between ideas is severed and the association of people limited, such that a task is mechanised and made routine in isolation, then cultures tend to develop where people become protectionist and ideas stagnate. Cultures where people lose sight of the connections between the various aspects of healthcare seem to feature in those healthcare organisations that have failed (Arbuckle 2013).

Walker's moral model is particularly useful in considering children's nursing because of the various groups who participate in it as discussed in Chapter 4 (child, carers, nurses, organisations, communities). Using Walker's model, the different views of children, their carers and nurses would all be valued and the interactions between them considered and critiqued. Who takes responsibility or avoids taking responsibility *for* children's nursing, well-being and health would then be negotiated between the parties.

What neither a pragmatic approach nor Walker's morality can offer is any certainty as to a right or proper way to do children's nursing. As Rorty (1996b) has pointed out, some may find pragmatists a little annoying, in that they offer rather vague contextual hedging instead of a prescription for how to do things. Some children's nurses may prefer the clear-cut morals of a quasi-religious or religious vocation devoted to children as innocents, defended by nurses as children's saviours in a world of adult agendas (Carter 2009).

Two points are worthy of consideration. First, while a dogmatic certainty would privilege one group, it would be at the cost of others. In the example above, nurses may achieve a comforting certainty by using their faith on which to base their nursing, but this does not allow a space for the views of children or of their carers, who may have other religious beliefs or no faith. Obviously it also alienates nurses who do not share a faith-based approach. Second, a pragmatic approach to children's nursing does not necessarily have to result in a relativist quagmire.

There may be points of disagreement about how children living with illness are to be treated, but in many communities there is also much agreement about how children should live a childhood. Children and their childhoods tend to be something about which people in communities care, particularly parents (see mumsnet.com/campaigns). Matters affecting children are often highly emotive and highly politicised. In an evolutionary sense, it would seem important that any community secures the well-being of its children, at least until they reach sexual maturity, otherwise it may cease to exist as a community. What pragmatics offers is a process, rather than a prescription. In any and all times, in any and all cultural spaces, using Walker's morality and a pragmatic approach allows us to gather the parties together, to acknowledge the conflicts and the points of agreement and to negotiate a consensus.

Any negotiated consensus involves parties giving up aspects which they may hold in high regard: nurses might have to give up some power, children may have to give up being looked after to take on more self-care and children's carers may have to give up some control to allow nurses to care for their child. As David Graeber (2013) has discussed, consensus may take longer and is more difficult to achieve, but in any situation where a vote is taken decided on the majority prevailing, there will be a minority who feel aggrieved. A minority who may continue to harbour resentment and who may not support the majority decision. In delivering healthcare, not having everyone on board can be very damaging. We know that if people think an intervention will work, it is more likely to do so, and in addition, if they think their clinician thinks the intervention will work, it is much more likely to be effective just from the placebo effect (Goldacre 2008). Even passive non-acceptance can influence the delivery of care. Consider the child who resists having blood taken. The nurse, the child's carers and the clinical team all agree blood needs to be taken – the child is a minority of one. The child's resistance may take many forms – hiding, crying, etc. – rarely does it involve verbal reasoning. The child may be held and blood taken forcibly, but each time blood is required the child is traumatised, their carer is traumatised, the nursing staff are stressed and in addition the process takes a great deal of time and often additional staff. Some clinical teams use a child-focused approach to gain the child's consensus. This takes time and expert intervention, but over time children learn to cope with the discomfort and become more active in the process, reducing and eventually removing the need to forcibly take the blood (Randall and Hallowell 2012).

There are two issues raised in Chapter 4 to which I want now to return. They are related and have ethical dimensions which it is important to consider here. In the negotiation of responsibility and avoiding responsibilities in children's nursing, nurses and children's nursing has a considerable advantage. Nurses are employed by organisations and are members of a regulated profession. As employed professionals, nurses have a vested interest in what Abbott and Meerabeau (1998) call social closure: the ability to limit the work of, in this case, children's nursing to a prescribed group. In order to work as a children's nurse, one has to obtain certain educational standards first to enter nursing programmes and then as a part of the programme that leads to a qualification which is a prerequisite to registration, which is required to gain employment as a children's nurse. The education qualification differs between states and for different types of nursing registration within states, but the principle remains. Some people are excluded from the work of children's nursing, while others are permitted to undertake this work. In most states children's nursing as a specialist qualification or category for nurse registration does not exist, but the same process applies to nurses who are seen as generalists (adult) nurses and who work with children. The process is controlled in states by the use of the legal system. Thus social closure in nursing is achieved through both education and legislation. The legal system can also be used to impose the clinical teams' view on children and on their carers. Case law in various states indicates that the state will normally take the side of the clinician over that of either children or their carers (Cantor 2005). Power then is not equally distributed in the negotiation of who is able to accept and reject responsibility *for* nursing children.

Social closure may be tolerated in communities because professions, according to Abbott and Meerabeau (1998), also promise to fulfil a social contract. In exchange for the income and social standing that employment and professional status confer, children's nurses are expected to deliver nursing care to children. Parsons' (1951) work on the sick role suggests that the professional in the sick role relationship is expected to be competent, accessible, altruistic and selfless.

There are, however, some challenges to the social closure/contract of professional employment posed by nurses facilitating children's childhoods. As was made clear in Chapter 2 childhood is relational. In Chapter 3 it was suggested that nurses needed to facilitate the care of children by their carers in order to sustain and develop the relationships between children and their carers as a part of the child's experience of childhood. In addition, a part of childhood is also the increasing independence children acquire as they progress with their peers to adulthood. Attempts to exclude the child's carers or even the child themselves from taking on the work of nurses contradicts the purpose of children's nursing to facilitate children's childhoods. Since requiring a nurse is not a part of childhood, and is stigmatised, it can be argued that the aim of nurses should be to make themselves redundant. Ideally the nurse should aim to have the child's carer or children themselves deliver their own care, to cope with illness with support of their family, friends and community, but not to be reliant on nurses. This aim of self-care or parental care is directly contrary to nurses achieving professional social closure.

Of course in most circumstances neither the child nor their carer can fulfil all the functions of the nurse, hence the need to have nurses. A solution to these conflicting dilemmas may be to recast children's nursing as work, rather than as a profession or a practice. Liaschenko and Peters (2004) have argued as much for nursing more generally. Work they argue can be undertaken by anyone with the required understanding and skills to perform the work to an agreed standard. As suggested by Walker's expressive collaborative morality, whoever accepts responsibility for aspects of the work or avoids taking responsibility can negotiate between the parties involved. Each party can express their view about undertaking the work, and the competency of the person undertaking the work can be assessed according to agreed standards and outcomes by agreed assessors. The understanding and skills that each party brings can be recognised. The circumstances under which another party might take responsibility for an aspect of the work can also be agreed, all without reference to educational and legal restrictions.

Accepting Walker's moral approach and the pragmatic approach requires a move away from professional and employment practices which restrict who accepts responsibility for children's nursing, towards understanding children's nursing as work which can be negotiated between children, their cares, nurses, organisations and communities.

Summary

The pragmatic approach does not offer a right and wrong morality to prescribe how nurses should deal ethically with children. Instead it offers a much more complex, challenging but ultimately more satisfying process of negotiation. Through Walker's expressive collaborative morality, all the voices in children's nursing can be valued. The power relationships between the parties can be recognised and who accepts or refutes responsibility for aspects of or the entirety of children's nursing can be negotiated. This negotiated pragmatic process allows for a critical exploration of the ethics of children's nursing within the context of a time and cultural/political space. Via such a process it can be determined who children's nursing works for and in what terms. Whether people in communities are satisfied with these arrangements is a political matter, action can be taken by them to challenge and change who children's nursing works for and the terms of what a community wants from its nurses and for its children. What pragmatics allows is for all the voices to be uncovered, for the positions of all parties to be considered and for a conversation to begin.

References

Abbott P and Meerabeau L (1998) Professionals, professionalization and the caring professions. In Abbott P and Meerabeau L (eds) *The sociology of the caring professions*, 2nd edn (pp. 1–19). London: UCL Press.

Admi H (1995) 'Nothing to hide and nothing to advertise' managing disease related information. *Western Journal of Nursing Research*, 17(5), 484–501.

Arbuckle GA (2013) *Humanising healthcare reforms*. London: Jessica Kingsley.

Bauman Z (1993) The moral party of two. In Bauman Z (ed.) *Postmodern ethics* (pp. 82–109). Oxford: Blackwell.

Blackford H (2004) Playground panopticism: Ring-around-the children, a pocket full of women. *Childhood*, 11(2), 227–49.

Cantor NL (2005) The bane of surrogate decision-making defining the best interests of never competent persons. *Journal of Legal Medicine*, 26(2), 155–205. doi: 10.1080/01947640590949922

Carnevale FA (2007) Revisiting Goffman's stigma: The social experience of families with children requiring mechanical ventilation at home. *Journal of Child Health Care*, 11(1), 7–18.

Carter B (2009) Tick box for child? The ethical positioning of children as vulnerable, researchers as Barbarians and reviewers as overly cautious. *International Journal of Nursing Studies*, 46(6), 858–64. doi: 10.1016/j.ijnurstu.2009.01.003

Christensen P and Prout A (2002) Working with ethical symmetry in social research with children. *Childhood*, 9(4), 477–97.

Corsaro WA (2011) *The sociology of childhood*, 3rd edn. Thousand Oaks, CA: Pine Forge Press/Sage.

Department of Education and Skills and HM Treasury (2007) *Aiming high for disabled children: Better support for families*. Norwich: Office of Public Sector Information.

Department of Health (2002) *Listening, hearing and responding*. London. Stationery Office.

Dewey J (1944) *Democracy and education: An introduction to the philosophy of education*. New York: Free Press/Simon & Schuster.

Finch Group (2013) Accessibility, sustainability, excellence: How to expand access to research publications report of the working group on expanding access to published research findings. Retrieved 17 August 2015 from www.researchinfonet.org/wp-content/uploads/2012/06/Finch-Group-report-FINAL-VERSION.pdf

Freidson E (1970) *Profession of medicine: A study of the sociology of applied knowledge*. New York: Dodd, Mead and Co.

Goldacre B (2008) The placebo effect. In Goldacre B, *Bad science* (pp. 63–85). London: Fourth Estate/Harper Collins.

Graeber D (2013) *The democracy project: A history, a crisis, a movement*. New York: Spiegel & Grau/Random House.

Kearney PM and Pryor J (2004) The international classification of functioning, disability and health (ICF) and nursing. *Journal of Advanced Nursing*, 46(2), 162–70.

Khair K, Meerabeau L and Gibson F (2013) Self-management and skills acquisition in boys with haemophilia. *Health Expectations: An International Journal of Public Participation in Health Care and Health Policy*. doi: 10.1111/hex.12083

James A, Jenks C and Prout A (1998) *Theorizing childhood*. Cambridge: Polity Press.

Liaschenko J and Peter E (2004) Nursing ethics and conceptulisations of nursing: Profession, practice and work. *Journal of Advanced Nursing*, 46(5), 488–95.

Mayall B (2002) *Towards a sociology for childhood: Thinking from children's lives.* Birmingham: Open University Press.

Murphy PJ (1990) *Pragmatism from Peirce to Davidson*. Boulder, CO: West View Press.

Parsons T (1951) *The social system*. London: Routledge and Kegan Paul.

Rorty R (1996a) Wild orchids and Trostky. In Rorty R (ed.) *Philosophy and social hope* (pp. 3–22). London: Penguin.

Rorty R (1996b) Introduction: Relativism: Finding and making. In Rorty R (ed.) *Philosophy and social hope* (pp. xvi–xxxii). London: Penguin.

Randall D (2011) 'To be like the others': Children's views of nursing in community settings. In Brykczynska G and Simons J (eds) *Ethical and philosophical aspects of nursing children and young people* (pp. 77–87). Oxford: Wiley-Blackwell.

Randall D and Hallowell L (2012) 'Making the bad things seem better': Coping in children receiving healthcare. *Journal of Child Health Care*, 16(3), 305–13. doi: 10.1177/1367493512443907

Randall D, Munns A and Shields L (2013) Next steps: Towards child-focused nursing. *Neonatal, Pediatric and Child Health Nursing*, 16(2), 15–20.

Randall D, Williams R and Wagstaff C (2010) The parent trap: Promoting poor children's mental health. *Poverty. Journal of the Child Poverty Action Group*, 137(Autumn) 11–15.

Royal College of Nursing (2010) *Restrictive physical intervention and therapeutic holding for children and young people: Guidance for nursing staff*. London: Royal College of Nursing.

Salinas E (2007) *Evaluation study of the staying positive pilot workshops: A self management programme for young people with chronic conditions*. Oxford: Expert Patient Programme, University of Oxford.

Sheehan T (1988) Heidegger and the Nazi. *New York Review of Books*, 35(10), 16.

Walker MU (2007) *Moral understandings: A feminist study in ethics*. New York: Oxford University Press.

World Bank (2015) Data: Population ages 0–14 (% of total). Retrieved 22 February 2015 from http://data.worldbank.org/indicator/SP.POP.0014.TO.ZS

6 Worked example case studies

Introduction

One of the techniques used in concept analysis is to describe exemplar cases (Welch 2008). The point being that in an exemplar case one can explore a nuance of the concept, adding detail and exploring themes in more depth. Hopefully in a way that makes the concepts seem more real, and more relevant to the practice of children's nursing, in this case. The point of these cases is not to describe all the nursing care in great detail, but to discuss how each case reveals and relates to aspects of the pragmatic children's nursing theory as set out in this book.

The cases in the chapter are not descriptions of actual people, or events. In a sense they are composites drawn from over 20 years of practice as a children's nurse, and from over a decade of teaching children's nursing. I have used such scenarios in teaching and research projects previously (Shaw et al. 2014). One of the challenges of such fictional accounts is that it is impossible to provide the degree of data which we as humans absorb from our empirical experience of events. All such cases lack the sort of detail which one would find in an account of events that someone has experienced, what Geertz (1975) termed 'thick description'. The use of vignettes or scenarios can also suffer from 'metaphor die back'. They are constructed to be illustrative, but if the reader takes them too literally, then the point can become lost. One can use metaphor in teaching to illustrate a point, this can be a very powerful tool as humans like stories and are programmed to responded to them (Beverley 2000). Unfortunately, people can like the stories too much: they latch on to the metaphor and become interested in exploring the metaphor. In using metaphor, we are saying that the concepts are like something else, they are not the something else, but are like it. The problem comes if one explores the metaphor too much and ends up at some point discussing the differences between the chosen metaphor and the context, rather than focusing on the illustrative point. Pushed far enough, most metaphors, if not all, fall apart.

With these limitations in mind I want to set out four cases. In part because this book is speculative, pragmatic children's nursing is a proposal and we therefore do not have empirical accounts to draw on, albeit that some elements of what is set out in this book are already present in children's nursing practice and literature. A coordinated and theoretically coherent pragmatic approach remains a proposal. It should of course be the aim of children's nursing researchers to evaluate the implementation of the pragmatic children's nursing approach should it be adopted in practice, so that, in time, we might replace these fictional accounts with empirical data.

I have chosen to construct cases from acute, long-term, community-based care and from palliative care settings. This is not to suggest that these encompass the totality of children's nursing, but merely to offer some breadth and depth of analysis in different illustrative settings. The cases are relatively simple. In reality more often than not there would be at least one if not more complicating factors. However, experience over the years has lead me to believe that children's nursing is highly complex and that even very simple cases hold more complexity than is helpful for illustration.

Each case is described briefly and then explored using the outcome measures set out in Chapter 3 and the educational process described in Figure 3.1. A reference table of these outcome measures is presented in Box 6.1 with a reproduction of Figure 3.1 in Figure 6.1. The outcome measures are often referred to in parentheses in an attempt to show how the outcome measures link to the plan of care (e.g. 'The nurse will need to assess Erin's capacity to meet Alan's needs as he undergoes surgery and recovers (3.5)').

Box 6.1 Outcome measures for pragmatic children's nursing

Outcome measure	Description
3.1 Health	Extent to which nurses are able to promote, restore and stabilise health status which allow children to participate in their childhood, with their peers in their communities.
3.2 Participating in a childhood	Number of days/occasions children are away from the environments in which they would access their childhood with their peers in their communities; for example, missed school days.
3.3 Self-care	Nurses can demonstrate how they • assess and reassess children's capacity to self-care • developed children's skills and understanding to facilitate self-care • encourage and facilitate children to be active partners in their own care.
3.4 Negotiating care	The nurse has a negotiated plan of responsibilities for aspects of care where the child, their carer and the nurse all have defined and agreed responsibilities in the plan of care. This plan of responsibilities is regularly reviewed and revised.
3.5 Supporting children to live a childhood	Nursing care plan demonstrates understanding of the • child's position in their childhood • parent's capacity to meet the child's needs and the skills or understanding that carers/parents need to develop to meet the child's needs • illness process and how it may affect the child and their childhood. Where possible the child's main carer feels competent and confident to deliver care and care is delivered by the child's main carer to a proficient standard.

Outcome measure	Description
3.6 Safe care	Nurses ensure the safe delivery of care to children including, when appropriate, preventing a child's carers from delivering care if it can be established that
	• through the actions of the carer the child is likely to suffer significant avoidable harm • programmes to facilitate the carer acquiring the required skills, attitudes and understanding have failed.
	Nurses act to make appropriate referrals to other healthcare and social care professionals and to work with others and carers to develop the carer's capacity to care for the child, either independently or with assistance.
3.7 Evidence-based care	Nursing care plan draws on current understandings of childhood, parenting, health and social care which are evidence-based, with identifiable and accessible sources. Nursing care reflects the time and space in which children are living their childhoods in their communities, with their peers.

3.8 Culturally safe care	The child and their carers feel respected as individuals from a particular cultural background.
	    Nurses are aware of and sensitive to different cultural practices related to children, childcare and health.
	    Nurses are able to challenge cultural practice if it can be demonstrated that the practices either adversely affect children's rights in relation to health and healthcare or the practices undermine other aspects of children's nursing interventions.

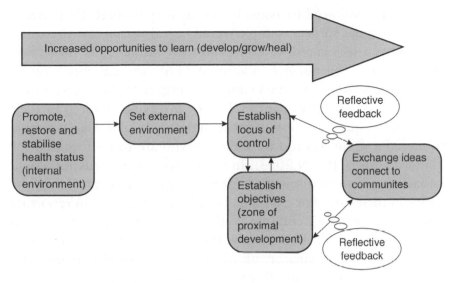

Figure 6.1 The pragmatic education process in children's nursing

Alan

Alan is six and has had repeated throat and upper respiratory infections over the past year. He is admitted for tonsillectomy and adenoidectomy under a general anaesthetic. Alan is an only child and lives with his parents. Apart from his throat and respiratory infections, which were treated with oral antibiotics, Alan has no other health problems. He attends his local primary school. His mother Erin is staying with him during his admission.

Plan of care for Alan

Alan is to be admitted as a day case, with the option to stay overnight if required. Using a pragmatic approach, the admission process would focus on Outcomes 3.2–3.5 and 3.7. The admitting nurse would need to welcome Alan and Erin, but focus on how Alan's repeated infections were affecting his integration into primary education. This is both about how Alan is coping with making friendship networks at school and about the impact that the infections may have had on his language development. The nurse is evaluating how the illness is affecting Alan's experience of childhood (3.5) of integrating with his peer group as they start their education.

The nurse will need to assess Erin's capacity to meet Alan's needs as he undergoes surgery and recovers (3.5). If we assume that Alan presents as a well cared for child and there are no child protection concerns that the nurse is aware of (3.6), we can move on to consider how Alan, the nurse and Erin negotiate their roles in the pre- and post-operative care (3.3, 3.4). Involving children in their care is not a quick process and it would be helpful if Alan was able to attend a group session for children who are to be admitted for planned surgery (RCN 2013). In such a session a discussion could be facilitated which allowed children to explore how they might be active in their care. For example, by taking a lead in pain reporting – instead of waiting, children could tell the nurse they have pain and the nurse would look at how they could reduce the pain. This might lead to a discussion of ways children could manage pain themselves; for example, distraction by playing a game, watching TV, etc. If Alan had accessed the group preparation, the admitting nurse could check his understanding and agree common strategies. Using the idea of ethical symmetry, Erin as Alan's mother could be offered a similar group session for children's carers. It is often helpful to have separate group sessions for children and adults that run in parallel and then come together for a short period. Illness and other commitments may make it difficult for children and their carers to attend pre-surgery sessions, so in any event the nurse will have to evaluate Alan and Erin's understanding of the proposed procedure and associated pre- and post-operative care, negotiate how child and mother are to be involved, and assess what responsibilities they themselves as the nurse (or the nursing team) are accepting. A standardised care plan might be used to outline the responsibilities that would be normally expected in such a case as in Box 6.2.

Box 6.2 Tonsillectomy and adenoidectomy care plan: day case admission responsibilities accepted

During your stay on the ward your nurse will:

- Answer any questions
- Tell you about things before they happen
- Help you to keep in contact with your friends and family

Before your operation the nurse will:

- Show you the ward area and introduce you to other children who are staying on the ward
- Show you where the play area is and how to get toys and other things to play with during your stay including how to use the TV and games consoles
- Check your health before your operation (test blood pressure and temperature and other things as needed)
- Help you to get ready for your operation (perhaps to get washed and put on your gown, remind you to go to the loo!)
- Make sure you have all the documents you need for your operation and that you are going for the right operation
- Help .... [insert name of carer] to support you as you get ready and go for your operation

After your operation the nurse will:

- Make sure you are safe as you wake up and get back to normal
- Check your health (take your pulse, blood pressure and temperature)
- Tell your doctors about how you are getting on
- Help you to manage your pain by giving you medicine and in other ways
- Make sure you have had something to drink, played if you want to and been to the loo (for a wee) before you go home
- Talk to you and .... [insert name of carer] about what to

do and what not to do when you leave the ward, get home and when you go back to school/playgroup

- Give you any medicine you need to take home
- Tell you and .... [insert name of carer] about when and where you may need to come back to see your doctor

During your stay you agree to try to:

- Talk to the nurse about your family, friends and your school so they can get to know you and about your health
- Let the nurse check your health and help you get ready for your operation
- Tell the nurse if you feel ill or have pain
- Let the nurse or .... [insert name of carer] know if you are hungry or thirsty
- Share the TV, games and books on the ward with other children
- Not go in the parents' room so mums and dads can have some time to themselves
- Help .... [insert name of carer] to look after you in the ward

During .... [insert child's name] stay on the ward I agree to:

- Answer questions that help people understand about me, ... [insert child's name] and their health
- Help .... [insert child's name] to stay in contact with their friends and family
- Support .... [insert child's name] before and after the operation
- Let the nurse know if I feel .... [insert child's name] is in pain
- Help .... [insert child's name] to cope with their pain by perhaps distracting them by playing a game
- Talk to nurses about my concerns
- Listen to what the nurse has to say about medication and

what to do or not to do on returning home and discuss what
I need to do to help .... [insert child's name] recover

After we go home I agree:

- To contact the nursing staff if I am concerned about ....
  [insert child's name] health and or recovery
- Follow the advice given by the healthcare staff on what to do
  or not do on returning home and when .... [insert child's
  name] goes back to school/playgroup

Delete sections, words as appropriate

Signed .... date ....

Signed .... date ....

Signed .... date ....

The language used here may seem oversimplified but we should
remember that the commitment to a pluralist view taken by pragmatists involves nurses making their work accessible to other parties. If
all parties views are to be valued and negotiations conducted between
all parties involved in children's nursing, then we as nurses have to
engage as wide an audience as we can by using very simple language,
by being prepared to discuss what we do and by being creative about
how we engage people with communication difficulties.

I want to turn now to how the plan of care for Alan might fulfil
the process of education/healing set out in Figure 6.1. Making
a space to discuss the responsibilities is also setting the locus of
control (Figure 6.1): setting out agreed responsibilities determines
who is controlling which aspects of the work. In the case of Alan,
we might suggest that the nurse is responsible for Alan's safety

during his stay, while he and Erin are in control of communicating how he is feeling. These are two examples, we could draw up a long list, but these seem reasonably obvious from the information in Box 6.2. In Alan's case we might suggest that much of the external environment is determined by the hospital as an institution, the structure and layout of the ward, the passageways to the operating theatre, how the theatre suite is set out, its staffing levels, etc. Of course within certain boundaries environments can be changed. Thinking about the environment might lead nurses to change practices in order to allow Alan and Erin privacy as they discuss his admission and health. A side room might be used as an interview space rather than a bed space on the open ward. The admission will as stated also allow for discussion of Alan's expectations of the operation and his recovery, which is the construction of objectives for the admission. For example, Alan might be fearful about the level of pain and discomfort he will experience. His understanding about hospital operations may be informed by the cultural view of hospitals as places where people go to die and that nurses inflict pain on people. Part of the proximal development of his understanding might be to explore these conceptions and to discuss how some pain and discomfort might need to be endured to remove the infected tissue in his throat that has been causing him to be unwell. We should remember that children's conceptions of illness may differ from that of adults. Although as Raman and Winer (2002) have shown, adults and children share conceptual ideas about illness, children may be less likely to employ a technical rational approach based on biomedicine, and more likely to subscribe to folkloric or immanent justice approaches. We are considering here the case of Alan on an individual basis, but we should also remember he is part of a community. The perceptions of a hospital admission can be addressed on a population level by nurses being involved in the sort of group session described above for children being admitted or on a more general scale by being involved in communities and schools talking to children about their health and hospital services. A public health agenda for children should include education programmes which prepare children to cope with illness and to interact with healthcare workers in an assertive way, incorporating ideas used in adult medicine of the expert patient (Salinas 2007).

Such a programme would fulfil the aspect of communicating ideas in communities (see Figure 6.1).

We might hope that when Alan is admitted his internal environment is stable, that is, his health status is reasonably stable. We know he enjoys good health, apart from the frequent infections. Initial assessment of health status recording pulse, blood pressure and temperature, and subsequent assessments as he recovers would address Outcome 3.1. The point of nurses facilitating the practice of medicine – the scraping of infected tissue from the tonsil bed and removal of adenoids – is to facilitate Alan participating in his childhood, not having to miss school because of his repeated infections (3.2). Alan's plan of care needs to be understood within the context of current understanding about how repeated tonsillitis is treated (e.g. NICE pathway for ear, nose and throat conditions (NICE 2013)), fulfiling Outcome 3.7 for nursing care to be evidence-based. Part of critically evaluating the evidence base of nursing care for Alan should be the extent to which Outcomes 3.1 and 3.2 are met. Monitoring Alan's health status through his recovery should allow for the nurse to assess how well Alan is recovering his capacity to participate in his childhood. Controlling pain, encouraging play and education activities would all be included. A measure of the nursing care should be how many days Alan misses from school (3.2). By understanding the evidence base, nurses should be able to advise on a suitable return to school: returning too soon and being exposed to upper respiratory infections may lead to an infection in the healing tonsil beds, which can lead to secondary bleeding (Lewis et al. 2013). Although we are not considering Outcome 3.6 here in terms of child protection, having assessed that Erin is able to deliver safe care, we should consider how the nurse ensures safe delivery of care. Ensuring safety applies equally in the hospital setting as it does in the home and community, thus giving advice about avoiding infections is a part of meeting Outcome 3.6 as is taking appropriate steps to report potential risks from understaffing or the poor cleaning of equipment (NICE 2006).

Finally I want to consider cultural safety as outlined in Outcome 3.8. There are of course many aspects to undergoing surgery which may pose cultural challenges. Exposing one's body to strangers is taboo in many societies. While there may be a social acceptance of healthcare workers viewing the body in line with their work, being wheeled on a trolley in a surgical gown exposes the child to the gaze of just about anyone who is passing through the hospital corridors. Would it be so difficult to build operating theatres with pre-surgical areas where people could get changed and have their pre-medication in comfort? Although there is little empirical work on children's sexuality in the hospital setting (Popovich 2003), we should not underestimate the potential for nursing care to cause children embarrassment (Randall 2010; Randall and Hill 2012). One of the challenges of delivering culturally safe care is that what is culturally safe is determined by the person receiving care. Nurses have to listen to children individually and encourage them to express their fears in order to understand what may upset them and when. Cultural practices are enacted by adults as well as children. A common practice amongst some parents is not to tell children when they are returning if they have to be absent from the ward for a short period, reasoning that the child cannot tell the time, will be unaware of when the time has elapsed and will be upset by talk of the parent leaving. However, although I am unaware of any research evidence, my experience is that this ploy is counterproductive: it leaves children fearful that their parents may never return, uncertain and often very distressed. This practice may be a simple example from Outcome 3.8 where the nurse should challenge a cultural practice because disappearing without telling the child adversely affects the trust relationship between parent and child which is vital to their childhood.

In this very simple case of a common surgical procedure we can see that the aspects of both the educational process, set out in Figure 6.1, and the outcome measures reproduced in Box 6.1 interact, both within the process/measures and between these conceptual frameworks. In a pragmatic sense they form the multifactorial context of children's nursing which describes children's nursing in this case. There are no elements which are not used, and none which need to be added. As stated in Chapter 2 (p. 25), all the aspects of children's nursing are accounted for in our description. There is no Cartesian division between what children's nursing is and our description of it. So in this sense the pragmatic approach set out here works. With some luck it works to stop Alan experiencing repeated throat infections which will allow him to attend school and build his relationships with his peers, in his community. In addition it works to strengthen the relationship between Alan and Erin as child and mother.

Andrzej

Andrzej is admitted to the ward with a raised respiratory rate (43 per minute) and a 48-hour history of poor feeding. On examination he is tachypneic with a raised pulse rate of 170 bts per min. He is pyrexial (39°C) but his capillary refill time is normal (<2 seconds). He is three months old, breastfeeds, was born at term, had a normal delivery and has no postnatal complications or concerns. His mother Nikola has two other children aged 4 and 2 years old.

Plan of care for Andrzej

Using the outcome measures in Figure 6.1, care for Andrzej might focus on Outcomes 3.1, 3.2, 3.4 and 3.5 initially. The clinical picture given above might suggest Andrzej has bronchiolitis or at least some form of viral respiratory infection. It could be argued that as an otherwise well child he could be nursed at home by his parents/carers (Freeman et al. 2015). For now let us assume that this option has been considered by his medical team, but admission to hospital has been preferred. It should be remembered that although many infants deal well with bronchiolitis with very little nursing and medical intervention, others require ventilation and intensive care (Friedman et al. 2014).

If we start at the beginning of the pragmatic children's nursing 'educational' process (Figure 6.1), there is an obvious need to address Outcome 3.1 and to stabilise Andrzej's internal environment – his breathing, temperature and fluid/nutritional intake. The nurse may facilitate interventions to stabilise Andrzej's health status such as administering oxygen and paracetamol, but fluid and nutritional intake may require more negotiation. The nursing staff will need to ascertain how breastfeeding is progressing, but if we assume that Nikola is producing good volumes of milk and is keen to continue feeding, then stabilising Andrzej's intake is not only dependent on the actions of the nursing staff. If we refer back to Chapters 1 and

2 then continuing breastfeeding can be considered as a part of early experiences of childhood and the relationship between Nikola and Andrzej is integral to the experience of being breastfed (and of breastfeeding a child from the mother's perspective). Of course continuing to breastfeed is also supported by Outcome 3.7 because the evidence base for the benefits of breastfeeding children is substantial (WHO 2002). Arguably, a pragmatic approach to Andrzej's case demands that the stabilising of his health status is considered as a part of his experience of childhood and his relationships in childhood. So encouraging Nikola to feed Andrezj for short periods frequently will allow her to continue feeding, but restrict the volume of feed at any one time in his stomach – which will allow him to expand his lungs into his abdomen and aid his ventilation (see Page-Goertz 2015).

Many children's ward areas have informal and/or official policies to promote breastfeeding and to support women to breastfeed. What pragmatic children's nursing allows us to do is to place such policies into a theory for nursing practice, such that nurses can advocate for breastfeeding mothers to have private spaces in the hospital to rest, eat, drink and suckle their children. This is how nurses attend to the external environment, providing the environment to support and encourage breastfeeding which of course extends beyond the physical environment to the social and cultural environment as acknowledged in the UNICEF baby friendly scheme (see www.unicef.org.uk/BabyFriendly/).

However, the nursing staff will also need to assess Outcome 3.5, in particular Nikola's ability to care for Andrezj, as stress may affect breast milk production. Having Andrzej hospitalised and concern for her other children may affect Nikola's ability to breastfeed. The negotiation of care between nurses and mother (3.4) needs to account not just for Andrzej's needs but also for Nikola's breastfeeding needs. Some may say this is family-centred care. My argument would be that as children's nurses we are supporting Nikola to breastfeed because it furthers the outcome measures relating to Andrzej's childhood. Supporting Nikola to breastfeed stabilises Andrezj's health status (in the short and longer terms), it allows the relationship between mother and child to be continued, which influences the infant's experience of childhood (Mayall 2002), and it allows Andrzej to continue to experience breastfeeding as an infant. Rather than considering the needs of the family unit, as family-centred care would suggest, pragmatic children's nursing allows nurses to focus on the child's needs.

In Andrezj's case, the locus of control may rest with his mother and nurses, albeit that other family members may support Nikola in caring for Andrezj, and in her breastfeeding. The negotiation of care and the understanding of care goals will be between nurses and Andrezj's carers (more scenario D – shared understanding of nurses and carers; see p. 75). Which is not to underestimate the agency of infants expressed by cries and body language, but that nurses and carers need to take responsibility for Andrezj to construct care in Andrezj's interests, given that he does not have the verbal/social skills to express his own wishes (see ethical symmetries in Chapter 5). Obviously for Andrezj the consideration of 3.3 (self-care) will be limited by his capacities at this age.

As outlined in Chapter 3, and Figure 3.2, while nurses may have experience of nursing other children with bronchiolitis, there is an argument that in the negotiation of care (3.4) nurses need to be mindful of Outcome 3.5 in that Andrezj will remain dependent on Nikola assessing his health status and seeking medical assistance as appropriate (Kai 1996). Thus while nurses might be able to more quickly assess and intervene in Andrezj's medical care, the pragmatic approach suggests a more considered negotiation of care which seeks to increase Nikola's capacity to care for her child (3.5). This is not least because if Nikola's capacity to care for Andrezj during self-limiting illness of short durations (such as uncomplicated bronchiolitis, see Friedman et al. 2014) can be enhanced, he will require less hospitalisation (3.2), which in turn allows him to stay in his childhood environment, living his childhood.

Focusing on Andrezj's needs allows nurses to be mindful of Outcome 3.6 (safe care), while supporting breastfeeding is important as outlined above since some infants with bronchiolitis cannot sustain suckling and may require supplementary feeding either orally or via a nasogastric tube to maintain their oxygenation. Nikola may be resistant to supplementary feeding as it can disrupt breastfeeding to such an extent that re-establishing feeding may not be possible. This then brings us to the final element of pragmatic children's nursing: the exchange of ideas in a community. Breastfeeding has become a political issue (Smith et al. 2012) and removing the ability to breastfeed can be highly controversial and cause psychological distress. Nikola may be very resistant to giving up breastfeeding because of the beliefs and cultural identity that she assigns to breast-feeding and to being a breastfeeding mother. There is of course a cultural aspect to perceptions of breastfeeding which would relate to Outcome 3.8. Early referral to a breastfeeding advisor (or lactation consultant) may help to prepare Nikola for the possibility that she will not be able to continue feeding Andrezj.

Within health organisations a variety of cultural/political views will be evident on the issue of breastfeeding in public spaces. Some may support women breastfeeding, or more accurately the child's right to be fed! Others may object or obstruct efforts to facilitate breastfeeding. This is where the discussion in Chapter 4 of Bauman's ideas is useful for nurses to place their actions in the context of organisations, since the organisational support (or lack of it) for breastfeeding will directly impact on nursing practice. Nurses will need to engage with the '*them*' (hospital managers) on behalf of the '*thou*' (breastfeeding women). One cannot provide a private comfortable place for breastfeeding mother with access to good food and drinks without the support of the host organisation, or at least it makes it very difficult.

By adopting pragmatic children's nursing in Andrezj's case, we can see how through negotiating care with his mother and providing nursing interventions his health status can be stabilised and restored. Working through the education-based theory outlined in Chapter 3 allows the nurse to focus on the needs of Andrezj and to see the connections between the internal and external environment, as well as how negotiating the care locus of control and care objectives underpins the stabilising and restoration of health status. That in turn is influenced by ideas which are current in communities, in this case about breastfeeding and child health. All this is of course based on beliefs about the benefits of breastfeeding, including the extent to which children living with illness can or should be breastfeed, and these beliefs in a very real pragmatic sense influence nursing practice and nursing actions.

Angel

Angel is 11 and entering secondary education. She has type 1 Insulin Dependent Diabetes which was diagnosed when she was five. She lives with her mother, grandmother and six siblings in a mid-terrace house. Her mother works full time to support the family. At a recent clinic appointment Angel's urine was found to contain some glucose and her HbA1c result shows that her diabetic control has not been as good as her normal levels (HbA1c=12.1%). As her community nurse, you decide to visit her at home after school.

Plan of care for Angel

Children's nursing delivered in community settings presents some different challenges. The negotiation of responsibilities and the setting of the external environment are much more in the control of the child's carers and the child rather than the hospital or other healthcare facility institutional managers. It might be helpful to start, however, by considering Outcome 3.1. If we want Angel to discuss her diabetic control, she needs to have a stable health status. Her concentration will be affected if she has an infection or is hypo- or hyperglycaemic (Connolly and Kvalsvig 1993; Shehata and Eltayeb 2010). Assessing her health status and taking appropriate action will facilitate Angel's learning and increase the likelihood of eliciting a reasonable history in terms of her diabetic control. Often in a community setting such an assessment may be more reliant on observation than physical examination – it is less likely to consist of taking a pulse and more on observing Angel's behaviour, although a repeat urine test for glucose and a review of her blood glucose monitoring would be useful. While making observation of Angel, we should remember that the visit is taking place after school. Angel may be tired and looking forward to some time to do what she wants, so a nurse's visit and answering questions from an adult may not be welcomed. With this in mind and having established that her blood glucose is within normal limits, for her, and that she has no other health concerns that require immediate action, the nurse can move on to consider Outcomes 3.2–3.5. In considering these aspects, we might want to consider first the environment of care, then focus on the locus of control and the objectives of care (Figure 6.1).

In many education systems, moving from primary education to secondary involves moving school, often from a smaller school with an ethos of individual supportive care to a much larger school where independence in students is encouraged. For children living with illness, this transition often highlights underlying problems they face (Royal College of Nursing Children and Young People's Mental Health Forum 2008). The communication between child, their carers, their teachers and nurses may need to be renegotiated in a new school and with higher student to staff ratios communication can be challenging. It is common (in my experience at least) for children living with illness to experience difficulties with their health management in the transition from primary to secondary education (see Prout 1989 and Yadav et al. 2010). It is easy to imagine in a small primary school class that all the pupils would be aware of Angel's diabetes, often teachers talk to the class about such health issues and encourage the children to share their own health problems. The children often stay together as a class. The school is small. If Angel is feeling unwell, her class mates may notice, perhaps alert a teacher. Angel can go to the sick bay (often the school secretary) because of the lower staff to student ratio there is more chance the staff will know Angel, allow her to keep her insulin in the fridge and give her a quiet, private place to inject. Compare this with many large secondary schools. Pupils are often in separate classes for lessons based on streaming or subject choice; Angel may not see her form mates all day, or they may share some classes but not all. It is less likely her fellow students would spot when Angel may be becoming unwell as they share less time. Her teachers will change according to subjects, so again a certain amount of continuity over the day is lost. If Angel herself realises she needs some extra medication, she has to excuse herself from class, from a teacher she may be less familiar with. Often in the larger schools she has to find the sick bay. Because of the increased number of students, it is less likely the staff will know Angel well, often negotiating access to a fridge is not easy in large schools and finding a private space to inject can be impossible (children often use the toilets, which is unacceptable). In addition to the environment of the school in general, there are social pressures associated with moving into a large school. Some of Angel's peers will move with her from primary to secondary, but she will also have to deal with groups of peers who may not have had an opportunity to discuss health issues. Bullying is being addressed in many schools (Department for Education 2014), but children living with illness are at higher risk and much still needs to be done to promote tolerance and the valuing of difference. Understanding the environment of the school, Angel's experience of both primary school and her transition into secondary school is vital to understanding the issues which may be affecting her diabetic control. She may of course have settled very well into a welcoming school environment with her peers, but she may also be feeling uncomfortable, not raising health concerns and her diabetic control is suffering because she feels unable to use her normal coping methods. There may be other reasons for her change in diabetic control, such as changes in her home environment or in relationships, or hormonal changes as she grows – all of which need to be considered. The change to her school environment is one factor, but it may be an important factor. The change in school environment is of course a part of Angel's experience of childhood, and understanding these potential changes is a part of situating Angel in her childhood (Outcome 3.5).

Let us assume that the change of school is the root of the deterioration in her diabetic control. The nurse has to attempt to assess Angel and her carer's abilities to deal with these changes and to manage Angel's diabetes in the new context of secondary school. Part of the objective of care will be to keep Angel in school (Outcome 3.2). As Angel will have to live with her diabetes all her life, helping her to learn to adapt her self-management to new situations is a vital skill (new job, new relationships, new locations). Thus assessing her self-care capacity is vital to helping her develop skills for life (Outcome 3.3). Part of this assessment will be understanding how Angel views the objectives of her care and what her motivation might be for achieving good diabetic control. While the locus of control might be with Angel, considering her as a competent self-managing patient, like an adult, we also need to use ethical symmetry to understand how being a child might affect her self-care. In this case we need to assess how Angel's grandmother is able to support her. As her mother works full time, it is Angel's grandmother who is at home when Angel leaves and returns from school, so she is most likely to be able to remind Angel to eat and to monitor her blood sugar, and to support Angel in decision making on a day-to-day basis. Including Angel's mother is also necessary, as is considering the health of Angel's carers, as a part of assessing the support for Angel in managing her diabetes. The balance between meeting Outcome 3.2 and for filling 3.5 will be integral to Outcome 3.4. That is, the balance between self-care and carer's directed care (and the nurse interventions) have to be negotiated, and regularly reviewed. It may be useful to include in this teachers as carers of Angel. Thus the nurse may negotiate with Angel's teachers what responsibilities they are willing to accept.

Healthcare workers should remember that educators, while they have a duty of care to children, are not responsible for healthcare management, but educational progress. Teachers may have legal, unionised and personal justifications for not offering to support Angel. To outsiders these can seem officious and obstructive, but for teachers accepting responsibilities for one child can place them potentially in a very difficult position, which may even threaten their employment and/or the education of other children. Accepting responsibility for say reminding Angel to eat at lunch time could set a precedent and lead to demands for teachers to issue a range of health reminders to children with asthma, eczema and other conditions. The legal position if a teacher were to forget to perform these functions is unclear, as they are not healthcare workers and have not received education on being a healthcare worker. They may not be contractually obliged to provide this sort of support, and with their education workload it may not be unreasonable that they occasionally forget. Without the education on healthcare, they may not realise the implications of their actions (or omissions). This does not mean that nurses should not negotiate with teachers, just that they should be aware of the challenges and of the concerns teachers might have. Being aware that workers in other disciplines and agencies have other concerns and agendas which may conflict with children's healthcare concerns may apply equally to negotiating the acceptance of responsibilities with other children's workers such as social care or housing workers. With these points in mind, we might propose the framework in Box 6.3 for allocating responsibilities in Angel's case (we are here making some assumptions which would be dependent on the details of an actual case, e.g. Angel's range of blood glucose levels). Many of the aspects listed here might be in Angle's Education and Health Care plan (EHC) if she is a student in the UK (Department of Education and Department of Health 2014).

From the scenario we might assume that Angel's family are struggling financially, depending on the sort of employment her mother has secured, even so with seven children and one income they are likely to be living in poverty. The restricted family income may affect Angel's ability to self-care and her carers' ability to support her self-care. Outcome 3.6 might be used to consider this threat to the safe delivery of care. If we assume that there are no child abuse concerns, we may still consider poverty as a social neglect (Southall et al. 2003). A referral could be made to social care for assistance or to a non-profit charitable organisation who may assist with financial planning, low interest loans or providing essential items. There are funds and/or opportunities from groups such as Diabetes UK which may allow the family to take a holiday for example. While this may seem to be outwith nursing concerns, as I have already argued, a family holiday may be an important childhood activity. It may also be a cultural practice which, if the nurse can facilitate, will allow Angel to pass as a 'normal' child in her community. The work of passing for children living with a long-term illness such as diabetes is, as previously discussed, a vital part of accessing their childhood (Chapter 4). Poverty will make Angel's attempts at passing more difficult. As Wilkinson and Pickett (2009) point out, being considered of lower social status than other members of your community brings with it social stress which can lead to physical and psychological harm. If the social stress of poverty is exacerbated by long-term health concerns, it is easy to see that strategies to reduce the social stress can help people to cope with their long-term illness. A family holiday may help Angel to present herself as like her peers (Carnevale 2007; Randall 2011a) but the relief from day-to-day concerns may also allow Angel and her carers to continue to manage her diabetes. For these reasons, family holidays for these children should be considered a very worthwhile investment for communities as they may well avoid the child being hospitalised and in some cases more damaging breakdown of social support and higher risks of disability.

Box 6.3 Suggested outline of allocation of responsibilities: Angel, her carers, teachers and nurse

Angel's self-care

I agree to:

- Monitor and report my blood sugar levels as agreed with the diabetic team
- Test and report urine dip test as agreed with the diabetic team
- Follow diabetic dietary advice and advise others as to my dietary needs (including mum and grandma, school)
- To undertake moderate exercise as advised and to adjust my diabetic regime as required
- To administer my insulin as agreed with my diabetic team and as suggested by my blood and urine monitoring
- To safely administer my insulin and dispose of all needles, medicines and any other equipment
- To tell mum, grandma or my teacher if I feel unwell and let them know if I feel hypo-or hyperglycaemic
- To call .... [insert name of nurse] and discuss aspects of my diabetes or diabetes care which concern me

Angel's carer (mum/grandma)

We agree to:

- Remind Angel to eat, exercise and monitor her diabetes as per the advice from her diabetic team
- To provide safe storage for Angel's medication and equipment in the home and when she is away from home
- To ensure Angel has an adequate supply of her medication and equipment to manage her diabetes
- To supervise Angel's disposal of needles, medication and medication to ensure safe disposal
- To discuss with Angel's teachers aspects of her diabetic care which may affect her education

- To take Angel to ward X if her blood sugar is less than XX mmol/L or more than XX mmol/L or if in agreement with Angel, her diabetic team and the ward team Angel is unwell and requires a medical review
- To call .... [insert name of nurse] to discuss concerns about Angel's diabetes or diabetes care

Angel's teachers

We agree to:

- Provide Angel with a quiet and private place in school for her to administer her insulin and or monitor her blood sugar. With particular regard to the potential stigma associated with living with diabetes
- Provide suitable storage for Angel's insulin at school should this be required
- Provide a safe place for Angel to dispose of needles and other equipment or medication she may require for her diabetes
- Ensure Angel's teachers have .... [insert name of nurse] contact details and have opportunities to discuss their concerns with .... [insert name of nurse]
- Create opportunities for all staff to be informed about health conditions which affect children at school. In particular to be informed about signs of hypo/hyperglycaemia and action to be taken by school staff
- If Angel is unwell or has a blood sugar level of less than XX mmol/L or more than XX mmol/L, we will call her mother on .... [insert number]. If we remain concerned about Angel and/or are unable to contact her mother, we will arrange transport for Angel and a teacher/teaching assistant to ward .... [insert local details]. We will inform Angel's mother of our actions at the earliest opportunity
- Create opportunity for Angel and her peers to discuss health, healthcare and living with a long-term health condition which allows Angel, if she wishes, to disclose and discuss her

diabetes and diabetic care. In particular, to discuss action to be taken if Angel's peers are concerned about her well-being, i.e. reporting to a member of staff

Angel's nurse

I agree to:

- Help Angel with her blood and urine monitoring and make sure the record of these is provided to the diabetic team regularly and on request
- Agree with Angel what information I can tell her mum/grandma/teachers/friends
- Only discuss the agreed information unless I feel that Angel or another child would be harmed by not discussing concerns with others
- Listen to Angel and try to help her understand how children live with diabetes and encourage her to care for herself, including adapting diabetic management to her life style (within safe limits)
- Refer Angel to other people who might be able to help her with problems in a timely way as challenges arise
- Listen to Angel's mum/grandma and her teachers' concerns and with agreement discuss these with Angel
- Ensure Angel's mum and grandma are able to access an adequate supply of her medication and equipment to manage her diabetes
- Talk with Angel's GP and school nurse to ensure the general practice team and school nursing teams are aware of her diabetes and her diabetic care needs
- Ensure appropriate arrangements are in place to allow Angel to access the medical and diabetic teams on ward .... [insert local details] and at hospital .... [inset local details] as an in- or outpatient as required
- Provide information to Angel, her carers, peers and teachers on the signs and symptoms of diabetes, how to manage it in

> the community, and on how and when to secure assistance
> to ensure Angel's safety
> - Bring all parties together to review, revise or redesign Angel's
>   diabetic care as required

How poverty affects children living with long-term conditions
and concerns about how children are stigmatised by illness are
perhaps ideas which connect nursing with communities (Figure 6.1).
Integral to these concerns will be cultural expectations and practices
(Outcome 3.8). Children who live with diabetes often struggle with
feeling different, particularly around their need to inject themselves
(Lowes 2007). Addressing these cultural/social stigmata may be
considered nurses' work on both at an individual level, attempting to
ensure Angel feels comfortable at school and home in managing her
diabetes, and at a population level. In the UK, school nurses can be
involved in addressing the stigma associated with illness in children
as a part of public health initiatives particularly associated with
public mental health initiatives (Lowes 2007).

It perhaps goes without saying that this plan of care for Angel
draws on a wide evidence base (3.7). However, it is worth noting
that the research funding and focus remains more on the basic
science than on applied research on interdisciplinary efforts to help
children to live with diabetes. We do not know, for example, whether
if nurses work closely with schools to facilitate children living with
long-term conditions in schools, helping to design school environments and policies to support children, does in fact translate into
better self-management, and in the case of diabetes, in better diabetic
control (or not).

Alma

Alma is 15 and she has a large neuroblastoma occupying a space in
her temporal lobe. Her tumour is inoperable and her medical team
has decided not to offer further radio- and chemotherapy based
on the response of her tumour treatment and the side effects she
suffered. Her parents have asked to take her home, and palliative

care at home with support from a local children's hospice has been agreed. Alma has a brother Jamil who is 11. They live with their parents and uncle.

Plan of care for Alma

Back in Chapter 2 we considered the 'special' case of the dying child. In the case of Alma we are considering the educational process set out in Figure 6.1 as having value in and of itself rather than just in terms of facilitating children's progress to adulthood. From the scenario, it seems unlikely that Alma will reach adulthood (defined in Shaw et al. 2014 as aged 18 – see Spectrum of Children's Palliative Care). We might not be surprise if she died in the next few months (orange category in the Spectrum, Shaw et al. 2014). So in regard to Outcome 3.1, the nurse may not be able to restore health status, and even stabilising health status may be unrealistic. We should perhaps consider that a nurse also cannot prevent Alan from having a secondary bleed from his tonsil bed and it becoming a fatal haemorrhage, Andrzej from suffering a fatal respiratory collapse or Angel from falling into a hypoglycaemic coma and dying. However, the Outcomes in Box 6.1 should be considered in total and not one outcome measure isolated and made the arbiter of children's nursing quality. Each of the outcomes are subject to factors which are not in the control of the nurse – the child's capacity to self-care may be affected by learning difficulties, carers' abilities to deliver care may be affected by poverty and the generation of new understanding of children's healthcare and the distribution of this information may be underfunded and undervalued by communities. Nurses have to deal with the processes of disease and dying as they are in time and space, not unhappily as we might wish them to be. Thus children's nursing might aspire to Richard Rorty's (1982) limited aspiration for pragmatists of understanding how things hang together at this time.

In Alma's case, meeting Outcome 3.1 might be more about managing her symptoms to maximise her participation in her childhood against an inevitable process of dying. However, symptom management to allow her to interact with her peers and family is in itself important both for the relief of suffering and for the preparatory work of grieving (Goldman et al. 2006). These interactions with peers and family allow them to create memories which will assist them in grieving once Alma has died. Performing these 'normal' functions of a child can help children who are dying to feel in control when so many other factors in their lives are out of their control (the growth of the tumour, their failing body, the emotions of those around them). It is not uncommon for children to want to attend school or to sit exams, while realising that they will never use the qualification. Affording children an element of control is central to Outcome 3.3 and while often self-care in a pure sense may not be appropriate or achievable, encouraging participation in care should remain a goal, albeit one that is necessarily tempered by the process of dying, and the associated deterioration in physical and cognitive skills.

The desire to 'pass' can be just as strong in children living with a life-limiting condition as for other children living with illness (Grinyer 2012; Carnevale 2007; Randall 2011a). As discussed previously, 'passing' and access to the environments of childhood are closely linked. Just as for Outcome 3.1, the process of dying may make meeting Outcome 3.2 gradually less important, and in practical terms less achievable. The attempt at passing is not always possible.

A major challenge for nurses in delivering palliative and end of life care to children, such as Alma, is that the evidence base is at best nascent and often simply not developed at all (Craft and Killen 2007; Grinyer 2012). In attempting to meet Outcome 3.1 and manage symptoms there is a developing literature on managing pain, but little on managing nausea, exhaustion or anxiety (Wolfe et al. 2000; Goldman et al. 2006), and even less on what outcomes we should look for, how do we know what good children's palliative care looks and feels like? Which begs the question what is a good death in childhood? Thus setting the objectives for care (Figure 6.1) is somewhat controversial and challenging, albeit that often children and their carers set personal goals (Bluebond-Langner 1978; Bluebond-Langner et al. 2007; Welch 2008) for how the child wants to die. Delivering palliative and end of life care as per Outcome 3.7 which is evidence based is a challenge which nurses need to face and work to resolve. Nurses often working with others have started to attempt to fill in some of the gaps in our understanding (see together for short lives – www.togetherforshortlives. org.uk/professionals).

The spaces in which Alma is cared for (and is dying) would seem to have a major impact on the negotiation of who takes responsibility for Alma and for her dying (as a process). From the scenario we know that it has been agreed to deliver care in the home, with support from a local children's hospice. Often such support from a hospice would include respite care for Alma, access to various services for her parents and for Jamil, her brother. In palliative and end of life care, the environments in which dying for children is permitted and the ideas about dying in childhood in a community are strongly linked (Figure 6.1 environment and exchange of ideas to connect communities). The taboos which exist in many communities on discussing death, particularly death in childhood, and the cultural practices associated with death in communities can make access to hospice care a challenge. However, if children and carers can overcome initial concerns, or more accurately be helped to overcome social stigma which may be associated with using a hospice, then many families find such services and facilities to be very helpful in providing respite care (for preparatory grief work particularly with siblings) and providing a space for children to die which is not a hospital environment but is also not the family home, a space where the burdens of caring for a dying child (and the joy) can be shared. In addition, for many families the hospice can provide a space and prescribed times to grieve and to remember their child (annual celebrations days where families gather to remember and celebrate their children's lives). A children's hospice can allow carers and other family members to access a community of people who understand what losing a child is like, because they too have lived with the loss, albeit in different ways.

The involvement of hospice services in Alma's case does raise interesting questions about how responsibilities are negotiated. Children's nurses may be negotiating which responsibilities are to be met not just with Alma, and her carers, but also with other nurses in addition to other health, education and social care workers. The discussion in Chapters 4 and 5 on the nurse's relationship to organisations which deliver care might be useful to consider here. A hospice and particularly children's hospices are quite different organisations compared to state or commercial for-profit hospitals and community nursing services. They have very different foundation myths, missions and visions (Arbuckle 2013) which give rise to different cultures that affect care delivery and the interactions of the nurses who deliver care. For example, nurses in state nursing services may be somewhat envious of their colleagues in the hospice sector who can decide to take a child to the zoo for the day – such an action is common in hospice care, often well funded and supported by the organisation. Such a trip in many state-organised services would be seen as a waste of resources: the parent's duty, have to be risk assessed in triplicate, questions answered about staff insurance cover, transport is often not available and funding would often be difficult to secure. Alma's state community nurse may find it frustrating to attend the house for a planned visit to find she has been taken to the zoo for the day. Equally hospice nurses can find it frustrating that state services are inflexible and rule bound. We could of course have highlighted similar cultural clashes between Angel's community nurses and her hospital team. The point being that in palliative and end of life care the negotiation of responsibilities set out in Outcome 3.4 and implicit to the locus of control aspect of Figure 6.1 are complex and often emotionally charged.

The extent of self-care evident in palliative care may be less than in our other examples and may diminish. However, in all four scenarios there are occasions and opportunities for responsibility to be both taken away from children and to be taken for them (see Chapters 2 and 5). These issues are perhaps more easily seen but complex in the case of Alma, where the cognitive and physical capacity to speak for herself may diminish and could be absent as death approaches. The added complexity is that Alma's capacity to speak for herself will fluctuate, sometimes she may be very capable and insightful, at other times she may be comatose. Determining when to encourage self-care and when to negotiate responsibility for the child with the child's carers is, I think, a challenge for children's nurses. As yet I fear we do not have the tools to make such a determination as to whether a child is cognitively and ethically competent to make their own decisions on self-care. The design and validation of such a tool lies outside the scope of this book, but if children are not to be denied the opportunity to direct their own care and if their rights to such self-determination are not to be taken away from them arbitrarily, then a tool of capacity to self-care needs to be developed.

This will not be an easy task, but it is, I think, a required one. This is an example of how pragmatism leads to new questions, beliefs and actions. Determining the capacity of children to self-care is not easy because one has to pick out social construction of capacity, physical aspects, disease processes and understand the emotional labour of living with an illness in childhood. That is not to say that children's nurses are not deciding where to encourage self-care and where to negotiate responsibilities with carers each and every day because they are, it is just that currently I would suggest these decisions are based on intuition, experience and sometimes stereotypical views and prejudice (Randall 2011b). At best this makes nurses' decision making somewhat arbitrary – the decision is subject to getting a nurse with a certain set of experiences and good intuition – and at worst prejudicial – the decision may be based on certain views of a child's ethnic background or their family's social economic status.

Assessing the capacity of Alma's carers (her parents) to deliver care is also more challenging in palliative care with the added issue of grief and preparatory grief (Outcomes 3.4, 3.5 and 3.6). Tasks which one day the child's carer can perform competently and confidently may on another day be too difficult to perform. The emotional work of living with a dying child can interfere or simply the work of coordinating care can overwhelm carers. It may be wise for negotiations to include contingency plans for the times when the carers need a respite from caring and the nurse is required to assume the responsibilities of the carer. Although good communication strategies are useful, in that they may give carers agreed ways in which to say they want the nurse to take responsibility for an aspect of care, they are not always sufficient. The nurse's ability to observe and decide to offer, sometimes to insist, to take on a responsibility is vital. As is skill in taking responsibility for Alma in ways which do not undermine her relationships with her family, which are key to childhoods (particularly to short childhoods), and which also allow Alma's carers to maintain their confidence to care and not to feel isolated or pushed out. As suggested in Outcome 3.6, it may be helpful to enlist support and practical advice from other health and social care workers to aid Alma's carers to care for her. Psychological help may be useful as might financial advice and such support might be accessed through the hospice or independently.

Palliative and end of life care often requires long hours of care, sometimes at odd hours of the night, the emotional labour and the cultural construction of caring for the dying would all seem to make cultural sensitivity and safety particularly important in Alma's case (3.8). The expression of a religious faith and participating in religious practices at such times may be of importance to Alma and her carers. As discussed in Chapter 3, cultural sensitivity and cultural safety does not require an uncritical acceptance of all cultural practices. Nurses may well want to challenge the suggestion that life-threatening illness is a punishment or a trial in order to relive psychological suffering, particularly at the end of life and in grief work, especially in work with Jamil, depending on his conceptions of illness and death.

Summary

The case scenarios set out in this chapter have on purpose been kept as simple as possible; in practice, cases are likely to be more complex. Yet in each case all of the eight outcomes set out in Box 6.1 and all the elements of the process shown in Figure 6.1 have been clearly identifiable. Exploring these cases has made it clear that outcomes and the elements of the process interact not only with each other, but also between the outcomes and the 'educational' process (Figure 6.1). It is also clear that these are not linear schemas. In each case some outcomes appear in need of more urgent attention, and some aspects of the process appear to come to the fore. Thus while for Alan Outcomes 3.6, 3.5 and 3.1 are immediately important, for Alma 3.1, 3.4 and 3.8 might require more urgent focus. While for Angel the locus of control and environment aspects of the process (3.1) seem key, for Alan post-surgery stabilising of his health status is vital. All the elements are included, but not necessarily in the order which the diagrams presented here might suggest.

The inclusion of a case in which palliative and end of life care is required highlights how childhood is a process not just an end result. Childhoods need to be facilitated by nurses because childhood is important to children in and of itself not just as a passage to adulthood (James et al. 1998). Living a short childhood or one which might not result in entering adulthood is just as important as living one which forms part of a longer life as an adult.

Finally I think it is important to note how pragmatics in these cases has allowed us to explore the interplay of self-care by children living with illness and disability and the negotiation of responsibilities for children's health and access to their childhoods. The discussions have highlighted how disease process, and in some cases the process of dying, are as integral to understanding children's agency in their healthcare as is developmental processes. The cases also show the complexity for nurses of negotiating responsibilities for care not just with autonomous children and their parents, but also with other family members, teachers, hospice workers and social care colleagues. The recognition of the pluralist voices in pragmatics allows the nurse to consider all the parties involved.

References

Arbuckle GA (2013) *Humanising healthcare reforms*. London: Jessica Kingsley.

Beverley J (2005) Testimonio, subalternity, and narrative authority. In Denzin NK and Lincoln YS (eds) *The Sage handbook of qualitative research*, 3rd edn (pp. 547–57). California: Sage.

Bluebond-Langner M (1978) *The private worlds of dying children*. Princeton: Princeton University Press.

Bluebond-Langner M, Belasco JB, Goldman A and Belasco C (2007) Understanding parents' approaches to care and treatment of children with cancer when standard therapy has failed. *Journal of Clinical Oncology*, 25(17), 2414–19. doi: 10.1200/JCO.2006.08.7759

Carnevale FA (2007) Revisiting Goffman's stigma: The social experience of families with children requiring mechanical ventilation at home. *Journal of Child Health Care*, 11(1), 7–18.

Connolly KJ and Kvalsvig JD (1993) Infection, nutrition and cognitive performance in children. *Parasitology*, 107 suppl, S187–S200.

Craft A and Killen S (2007) *Palliative care services for children and young people in England: An independent review for the Secretary of State for Health*. London: Department of Health.

Department for Education (2014) Preventing and tackling bullying: Advice for headteachers, staff and governing bodies. Retrieved 17 August 2015 from www.gov.uk/government/uploads/system/uploads/attachment_data/file/288444/preventing_and_tackling_bullying_march14.pdf

Department of Education and Department of Health (2014) *Implementing a new 0 to 25 special needs system: LAs and partner duties and timescales – what you must do and when*. London: Department of Education and Department of Health.

Freeman JF, Weng HYC and Sandweiss D (2015) Outpatient management of home oxygen for bronchiolitis. *Clinical Pediatrics*, 54(1), 62–6. doi: 10.1177/0009922814547564

Friedman JN, Rieder MJ, Walton JM and Canadian Paediatric Society Acute Care

Committee and Drug Therapy and Hazardous Substances Committee (2014) Bronchiolitis: Recommendations for diagnosis, monitoring and management of children, one to 24 months of age. *Paediatrics and Child Health*, 19(9), 485–91.

Geertz C (1975) *Thick description: Toward an interpretive theory of culture. The interpretation of cultures: Selected essays by Clifford Geertz*. London: Hutchinson.

Goldman A, Hewitt M, Collins GS, Childs M and Hain R (2006) Symptoms in children/young people with progressive malignant disease: United Kingdom Children's Cancer Study Group/Paediatric Oncology Nurses Forum Survey. *Pediatrics*, 117(6), 1179–86. doi: 10.1542/peds.2005–0683

Grinyer A (2012). *Palliative and end of life care for children and young people: Home, hospice and hospital*. Chichester: Wiley-Blackwell.

Kai J (1996) What worries parents when their pre/school children are acutely ill and why a qualitative study. *British Medical Journal*, 313(7063), 983–6.

James A, Jenks C and Prout A (1998) *Theorizing childhood*. Cambridge: Polity Press.

Lewis SR, Nicholson A, Cardwell ME, Siviter G, Smith A and Cochrane Anaesthesia Group (2013) Non-steroidal anti-inflammatory drugs and perioperative bleeding in paediatric tonsillectomy. The Cochrane Collaboration. Wiley and Sons. doi: 10.1002/14651858.CD003591.pub3

Lowes L (2007) Impact upon the child and family. In Valentine F and Lowes L (eds) *Nursing care of children and young people with chronic illness* (pp. 55–83). Oxford: Blackwell Publishing.

Mayall B (2002) *Towards a sociology for childhood: Thinking from children's lives*. Birmingham: Open University Press.

National Institute for Health and Care Excellence (2006) IPG196 Patient safety and reduction of risk of transmission of Creutzfeldt-Jakob disease (CJD) via interventional procedures. Retrieved 23 February 2015 from http://guidance.nice.org.uk/IPG196/Guidance/pdf/English

National Institute for Health and Care Excellence (2013) Ear, nose and throat conditions pathway. Retrieved 23 February 2015 from http://pathways.nice.org.uk/pathways/ear-nose-and-throat-conditions

Page-Goertz S (2015) The ill child: Breastfeeding implications. In Wambach K and Riordan J (eds) *Breastfeeding and human lactation*, 5th edn (pp. 717–73). Burlington, MA: Jones and Bartlett Learning.

Popovich DM (2003) Preserving dignity in the young hospitalised child. *Nursing Forum*, 38(2), 12–17.

Prout A (1989) Sickness as a dominant symbol in life course transitions: An illustrated theoretical framework. *Sociology of Health and Illness*, 11(4), 336–59.

Raman L and Winer GA (2002) Children's and adults' understanding of illness: Evidence in support of a coexistence model. *Genetic Social and General Psychology Monographs*, 128(4), 325–55.

Randall D (2010) 'They just do my dressings': Children's perspectives on community children's nursing. Unpublished PhD thesis, University of Warwick, Warwick.

Randall D (2011a) 'To be like the others': Children's views of nursing in community settings. In Brykczynska G and Simons J (eds) *Ethical and philosophical aspects of nursing children and young people* (pp. 77–87). Oxford: Blackwell.

Randall D (2011b) Who is shaping children's nursing? In Brykczynska G and

Simons J (eds) *Ethical and philosophical aspects of nursing children and young people* (pp. 251–60). Oxford: Wiley-Blackwell.

Randall D and Hill A (2012) Consulting children and young people on what makes a good nurse. *Nursing Children and Young People*, 24(3), 14–19.

Rorty R (1982) Introduction: Pragmatism and philosophy. In Rorty R (ed.) *Consequences of pragmatism* (pp. xiii–xivii). Minneapolis: University of Minnesota Press.

Royal College of Nursing Children and Young People's Mental Health Forum (2008) *Lost in transition: Moving young people between child and adult health services*. London: Royal College of Nursing.

Royal College of Nursing (2013) Guideline 3: Day surgery information, children and young people in day surgery. London: Royal College of Nursing. Retrieved 17 August 2015 from www.rcn.org.uk/__data/assets/pdf_file/0009/78507/004_464. pdf

Salinas E (2007) *Evaluation study of the staying positive pilot workshops: a self management programme for young people with chronic conditions*. Oxford: Expert Patient Programme, University of Oxford.

Shaw KL, Brook L, Kaambwa C, Harris N, Lapwood S and Randall D (2014) The Spectrum of Children's Palliative Care Needs: A classification framework for children with life-limiting or life-threatening conditions. *BMJ Supportive and Palliative Care*, 5 March online first. doi: 10.1136/bmjspcare-2012–000407

Shehata G and Eltayeb A (2010) Cognitive function and event-related potentials in children with type 1 Diabetes Mellitus. *Journal of Child Neurology*, 25(4), 469–74. doi: 10.1177/0883073809341667

Smith PH, Hausman BL and Labbok M (eds) (2012) *Beyond health, beyond choice breastfeeding constraints and realities*. New Brunswick, NJ: Rutgers University Press.

Southall DP, Samuels MP and Golden MH (2003) Classification of child abuse by motive and degree rather than type of injury. *Archives of Disease in Childhood*, 88(2), 101–4.

Welch SB (2008) Can the death of a child be good? *Journal of Pediatric Nursing*, 23(2), 120–5. doi: 10.1016/j.pedn.2007.08.015

Wilkinson RG and Pickett K (2009) *The Spirit Level: Why more equal societies almost always do better*. Bristol: Allen Lane.

Wolfe J, Grier HE, Klar N, Levin SB, Ellenbogen JM, Salem-Schatz S, Emanuel EJ and Weeks JC (2000) Symptoms and suffering at the end of life in children with cancer. *New England Journal of Medicine*, 342(5), 326–33.

World Health Organization (2002) Infant and young child nutrition. Global strategy on infant and young child feeding. Geneva: World Health Organization.

Yadav V, O'Reilly M and Karlm K (2010) Secondary school transition: Does mentoring help at risk children? *Community Practitioner*, 83(4), 24–8.

Afterword

Once I had completed the first draft of this book, I started to share the ideas in the book. In this afterword I wanted to capture some of the initial reactions of people to the ideas. The first reaction, surprisingly, to me anyway, was that the theory was welcomed by clinical nurses. When I presented the ideas to senior clinical nurses, they recognised that they often did not have well-defined models or theories, that the ones they used were not adequate and that they needed to support their work with theoretical perspectives. I was perhaps surprised because I developed much of this work with students who were often less engaged with theoretical ideas and more with the 'doing' of nursing. The senior clinical nurses I have spoken with all recognised the problems of family-centred care and the inadequacy of current nursing models which use adult theories.

In our conversations, as I tried to explain the pluralism of pragmatics, an interesting idea was expressed by some senior nurses. If, as pragmatics suggests, there are many theories of children's nursing and all might be as valid, in that each might be 'good' in its own time and cultural social space and if this is accepted together with my assertion that there is no a theoretical position (Chapter 1), then does it not follow that each nurse might carry in their head their own theory of children's nursing and that might be ok! Essentially, that we already have pragmatic children's nursing, albeit in an uncritical form. There is already a plurality of children's nursing theories, each often unconsciously influenced and based on uncritiqued assumptions, which each children's nurse has built up over time, tested, refined and sculpted by practice.

This may well be the case. The more I worked on the book and the pragmatic ideas, the more I felt that it was not really an invention, but a discovery. That what I was setting out was not a new theory for children's nursing, but a drawing together of lots of aspects of children's nursing which I and my students and colleagues all knew well, but which lay disconnected and disparately about the field of children's nursing. Rather than being inventors in a laboratory, we might be more archaeologists uncovering children's nursing, the clues to which lay all about us and we had but to brush away the covering dust to see how the various aspects were connected together by the concept of living a childhood.

However, the concept of each nurse holding their own model or theory is problematic. First, there are challenges of conflicting beliefs within teams which might lead to conflicting actions of nurses. For example, one nurse might believe children should learn self-care from a young age, another might believe that self-care should not be expected until teenage years. So while one nurse teaches self-care, her actions could be undermined by another dismissing self-care as unnecessary (irrespective of the child's desires, or that of their carers). Second, this idea of individual theories feeds into a narrative where nurses state that each child is individual and that nursing can only be pursued in a case by case scenario. Of course each child is unique, but they are also children with specific health problems, living a childhood in a community and as such their nursing care will have common factors and aspects as well as individual features. The idea that a nurse should approach each child with an entirely blank page seems unrealistic, impractical and a waste of resources. Like going back to the drawing board every time one wanted to take a trip from A to B, moving between the points might be different each time with different weather and traffic condition, but we do not redesign the bicycle or car each time! Similarly nurses might hold different theories of children's nursing, but there will be a good number of common aspects to the theories. Hopefully all nurses might agree that play is important to all children. To ignore these commonalities and redesign care from scratch each time, not acknowledging any repeated features seems perverse, and wasteful of time, effort and resources.

The point of pragmatic children's nursing is to bring communities together to uncover the similarities and the differences in their understanding of children's nursing in order that they might deliver and receive more consistent, coherent and cognisant nursing care. Pragmatic children's nursing might evolve differently at different times in different cultural/social spaces, but it must be shared by communities. This point goes back to Quine's concept of *indeterminacy of radical translation* (Murphy 1990: 84; Chapter 2). The meaning of children's nursing occurs in a community; its meaning has to be shared by participants in that community. I include here children and their carer in these communities, not just professional nurses. The idea of individual nurses holding their own conception of children's nursing would not be pragmatic because the meaning is not shared between participants in communities. In addition, although pragmatic children's nursing might look and feel different in separated times and locations, it would still need to be based upon pragmatic ideas and concepts. Otherwise it would be another type of children's nursing. The different pragmatic children's nursing models would be bound together then by pragmatic children's nursing theory.

In my discussions with nurses about implementing pragmatic children's nursing, assessment of children's needs using the theory was a prominent concern. It seems unlikely that the pragmatic approach would alter the nursing process (Kratz 1979) of assess, plan, implement and evaluate to a great degree. Some aspects of the theory might draw on current assessment tools. The assessment of the internal environment could be undertaken using paediatric early warning scores or other physiological-based assessment tools (Parshuram et al. 2011). Nurses may wish to consider in light of the pragmatic children's nursing theory how new technologies might be used to enhance the assessment of internal environments and the indicators of internal environments which permit and promote participation in childhood activities, such as playing with peers. As discussed in Chapter 3, existing quality of life measures could be used to perhaps evaluate the effects of both internal and external environment, albeit that how such measures relate to experiencing a childhood needs to be established and validated.

The other aspects of pragmatic children's nursing will, I think, require new assessment tools. I am not aware of nursing tools to evaluate the effects on children's illness of external environments.

Again technologies could be helpful in providing feedback on environmental factors such as noise, light or ambient temperature, but would need to be augmented with nursing observation; for example, whether noise is causing the child distress or is the soundtrack of the movie *Frozen*! New tools will also need to be designed, developed, validated and evaluated to assess children's self-care, the balance of locus of control between children and their carers and the abilities of carers to provide care that promotes children's access to their childhood. There could be measures of fidelity with negotiated plans of care, that is, how well did children, their carers and nurses actually deliver the care they negotiated and planed (see Outcome 3.4). New ways to evaluate nursing care might assess the impact illness has on children accessing their childhoods. Simple measures might be counting the days, or opportunities children miss to engage in their childhood activities, be that school, college, sports clubs or other peer activities. A positive measure could be how nurses have facilitated children to interact with their peers. An entry in the nursing notes might read 'Encouraged James to text his best friend Paul who attended the ward. Boys played video games for 3 hours.' This could be part of a new index of childhood engagement factors which might include participation in education, play activities or interaction with peers. Measures and tools also need to be developed that would monitor safety of care, including cultural safety, to ensure minimum standards are consistently met and improvements tracked.

The degree to which care reflects the ideas of a community might need to be evaluated at a more strategic level, a more population basis, rather than on a case by case audit. This could include assessment of the degree to which care is evidence based. It should also feature public patient involvement in setting care agendas and in evaluating current provision. This assessment development programme is a demonstration of the way in which, as was stated in Chapter 2, pragmatics works as the beliefs about children's nursing give rise to doubt which in turn results in action. Here the pragmatic children's nursing theory raises doubts about how nurses assess children and that flows into a redesigning of assessment measures focused on how nurses facilitate children living with illness to live a childhood.

John Dewey wrote:

It is the very nature of life to strive to continue in being. Since this continuance can be secured only by constant renewals, life is a self renewing process. What nutrition and reproduction are to physiological life, education is to social life.

(1944: 9)

If the pragmatic children's nursing is to live as a social phenomenon, it must be open to constant critical appraisal. This may be the end of this book, but it is just the beginning of the work to research, validate or refute the ideas set out here – to create for each generation of children their own pragmatic children's nursing.

References

Dewey J (1944) *Democracy and education: An introduction to the philosophy of education*. New York: Free Press/Simon & Schuster.

Kratz CR (1979) *The nursing process*. London: Baillière Tindall.

Murphy PJ (1990) *Pragmatism from Peirce to Davidson*. Boulder, CO: West View Press.

Parshuram CS, Duncan HP, Joffe AR, Farrell CA, Lacroix JR, Middaugh KL, Hutchison JS, Wensley D, Blanchard N, Beyene J and Parkin PC (2011) Multicentre validation of the bedside paediatric early warning system score: A severity of illness score to detect evolving critical illness in hospitalised children. *Critical Care*, 15(4), R184. doi: 10.1186/cc10337

Index